T0113658

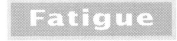

Fatigue

Fight It
with
the Blood
Type Diet®

DR. PETER J. D'ADAMO

WITH CATHERINE WHITNEY

Dr. Peter J. D'Adamo's

Eat Right 4 Your Type

Health Library

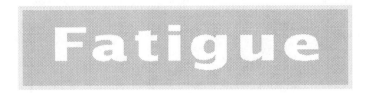

Fight It with the Blood Type Diet®

BERKLEY BOOKS

NEW YORK

THE BERKLEY PUBLISHING GROUP
Published by the Penguin Group
Penguin Group (USA) Inc.
375 Hudson Street, New York, New York 10014, USA
Penguin Group (Canada), 90 Eglinton Avenue East, Suite 700, Toronto, Ontario M4P 2Y3, Canada
(a division of Pearson Penguin Canada Inc.)
Penguin Books Ltd., 80 Strand, London WC2R 0RL, England
Penguin Group Ireland, 25 St. Stephen's Green, Dublin 2, Ireland (a division of Penguin Books Ltd.)
Penguin Group (Australia), 250 Camberwell Road, Camberwell, Victoria 3124, Australia
(a division of Pearson Australia Group Pty. Ltd.)
Penguin Books India Pvt. Ltd., 11 Community Centre, Panchsheel Park, New Delhi—110 017, India
Penguin Group (NZ), cnr Airborne and Rosedale Roads, Albany, Auckland 1310, New Zealand
(a division of Pearson New Zealand Ltd.)
Penguin Books (South Africa) (Pty.) Ltd., 24 Sturdee Avenue, Rosebank, Johannesburg 2196,
South Africa

Penguin Books Ltd., Registered Offices: 80 Strand, London WC2R 0RL, England

PRINTING HISTORY
G. P. Putnam's Sons hardcover edition / April 2005
Berkley trade paperback edition / January 2006
Berkley trade paperback ISBN: 978-0-425-20754-3

The Library of Congress has cataloged the G. P. Putnam's Sons hardcover edition as follows:

D'Adamo, Peter.
    Fatigue : fight it with the blood type diet / Peter J. D'Adamo with Catherine Whitney.—(Dr. Peter J.
    D'Adamo's eat right 4 your type health library)
        p.   cm.
    Includes index.
    ISBN 0-399-15254-7
    1. Fatigue—Diet therapy.   2. Blood groups.   3. Naturopathy.   I. Whitney, Catherine.   II. Title.
RB150.F37D33   2005   2004043156
616'.047—dc22

DEDICATED TO THOSE
WHO STRIVE TO LIVE FULLY
AND ENERGETICALLY
IN EVERY MOMENT

Acknowledgments

THIS BOOK OFFERS THE BEST THAT NATUROPATHIC MEDICINE and blood type science have to offer in overcoming fatigue. It has been a collaborative process, and I want to express my deep thanks to the people who have been involved in its creation.

I am most grateful to Martha Mosko D'Adamo, not only my partner in life and in parenting but also my partner in bringing the valuable wisdom about blood type to the world. Martha daily provides love, support, insight, and inspiration to all of my endeavors.

Catherine Whitney, my writer, and her partner, Paul Krafin, are invaluable word masters who have once again captured exactly the right tone in tackling this complex topic.

My literary agent and friend, Janis Vallely, always takes time to listen and advise. Her quiet guidance and personal support make the work possible.

I would also like to acknowledge others who have made significant contributions to the work: my colleague Bronner Handwerger, N.D., whose research and clinical abilities are invaluable; Heidi Merritt, who continues to make an important contribution to the work;

John Harris, whose knowledge and input have been invaluable; Laura Mittman, N.D., IfHI, who has been such a big help in my efforts to educate other professionals; and Catherine's agent, Jane Dystel, who provides crucial support.

Amy Hertz, my former editor at Riverhead/Putnam, was the force behind the blood type books. Denise Silvestro continues to shepherd the work with dedication and skill.

As always, I am extremely grateful to the wonderful staff at Riverhead Books and Putnam. They have been tireless and enthusiastic, and their efforts have made it possible to continue bringing this important work to the market.

PETER J. D'ADAMO, N.D.

Contents

Appendices

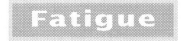

Fatigue

Fight It
with
the Blood
Type Diet®

New Tools to Fight Fatigue

THE BLOOD TYPE DIET CAN BENEFIT EVERYONE. YOU don't have to be sick to see the effects. But most of the people who come to my clinic or contact my Web site are dealing with a serious chronic disease or have received a distressing medical diagnosis. They want to know how they can hone the general guidelines of the Blood Type Diet to target their illness. Dr. Peter J. D'Adamo's Eat Right 4 (for) Your Type Health Library has been introduced with these people in mind.

Fatigue: Fight It with the Blood Type Diet allows you to take full advantage of the medicinal benefits of eating and living according to your blood type. If you think of the standard Blood Type Diet as the foundation, the guidelines in this book provide a more targeted overlay for people who experience deep fatigue, either as a primary or a secondary medical factor. These dietary and lifestyle adaptations, individualized by blood type, supply additional ammunition to fight fatigue, by strengthening your immune system and improving metabolic and cellular fitness.

Here's what you'll find that's new:

- A disease-fighting category of blood type–specific food values, the **Super Beneficials,** emphasizing foods that have medicinal properties to strengthen immunity, reduce stress, and address specific medical conditions that cause fatigue.
- A more detailed breakdown of the **Neutral** category to limit foods that are known to have less nutritional value. Foods designated **Neutral: Allowed Infrequently** should be minimized or avoided.
- Detailed supplement protocols for each blood type that are calibrated to support you at every stage. They include the **Basic Fatigue Protocol, Immune System Health Maintenance Protocol, Stress Management Protocol, Addressing Metabolic or Environmental Toxicities Protocol,** and **Cellular Blockage Protocol.**
- A **4-Week Plan** for getting started that emphasizes what you can do right now to improve your condition and start feeling better immediately.
- Plus many strategies for success, quizzes, checklists, and the answers to the questions most frequently asked about fatigue at my clinic.

The chemistry of blood type continues to provide important clues to the biological and genetic mechanisms that control health and disease. Increasingly, medical doctors and naturopaths throughout the world are applying the blood type principles in their practices, with remarkable results.

I urge you to talk to your physician about the benefits of incorporating individualized, blood type–specific diet, exercise, and lifestyle strategies into your current plan. I am confident that using the guidelines in this book will start you on the road to recovery. Take the step now, and use your blood type to your best advantage.

Why Blood Type Matters

YOU ARE A BIOLOGICAL INDIVIDUAL.

Have you ever wondered why some people are constitutionally frail and susceptible to infection, while others seem naturally hardy? Why some people are able to lose weight on a particular diet, while others fail? Why some people age rapidly and show early signs of deterioration, while others are full of vitality into their later years?

We are all different. A single drop of your blood contains a biochemical signature as unique to you as your fingerprint. Many of the biochemical differences that make you an individual can be explained by your blood type.

Your blood type influences every facet of your physiology on a cellular level. It has everything to do with how you digest food, your ability to respond to stress, your mental state, the efficiency of your metabolic processes, and the strength of your immune system.

You can greatly improve your health, vitality, and emotional balance by knowing your blood type and by incorporating blood type–specific diet and lifestyle strategies into your health plan.

Be the biological individual you were meant to be!

What's Your Blood Type– Fatigue Factor?

General Factors

THE FOLLOWING FACTORS are known to contribute to fatigue. Check yes for each question that applies to you, then total the values of the "yes" answers.

Risk Factor	Yes	Value
Are you menopausal?	☐	1
Do you have a history of following extreme, low-calorie diets, or of "yo-yo" dieting?	☐	3
Do you smoke?	☐	3
Do you average fewer than 8 hours sleep each night?	☐	2
Do you average more than 2 alcoholic drinks per day?	☐	1
Do you take medications for a chronic illness?	☐	2
Does your diet regularly include highly processed and frozen foods?	☐	2

Have you been diagnosed with chronic
fatigue syndrome? ☐ 3

Total the number of "yes" answer points (17 points maximum)

BLOOD TYPE–SPECIFIC QUIZZES

The Blood Type O Quiz

The following factors are known to specifically foster conditions of
fatigue for Blood Type O. Check yes for each question that applies
to you, then total the values of all "yes" answers.

Risk Factor	Yes	Value
Are you a non-secretor? (See page 21.)	☐	3
Do you regularly follow a high-carbohydrate diet?	☐	3
Do you have a history of depression?	☐	2
Do you consider yourself a "type A" personality?	☐	3
Do you suffer from hypothyroidism (low thyroid)?	☐	2
Are you susceptible to fungal conditions, such as candidiasis?	☐	1
Are you a vegetarian/vegan?	☐	3
Do you suffer from inflammatory problems, such as fibromyalgia or allergies?	☐	2
Is your level of aerobic exercise under 4 hours weekly?	☐	3

Total the number of "yes" answer points (22 points maximum)

Scoring: Total the values of "yes" answer points in both quizzes.

25–39: High to Very High Fatigue Factor. Take immediate action
with adherence to the Blood Type Diet, and modify the factors that are
in your control.

10–24: Moderate to High Fatigue Factor. If you make some diet
and lifestyle changes, you can minimize your fatigue factors. Refer to
your blood type section to determine which actions you must take.

1–9: Low to Moderate Fatigue Factor. Keep it that way by adhering to the Blood Type Diet and lifestyle plan.

The Blood Type A Quiz

The following factors are known to specifically foster conditions of fatigue for Blood Type A. Check yes for each question that applies to you, then total the values of all "yes" answers.

Risk Factor	Yes	Value
Are you a non-secretor? (See page 21.)	☐	3
Do you regularly follow a high-protein, high-fat diet?	☐	3
Do you spend more than 90% of your time in an urban environment?	☐	2
Do you eat red meat or dairy products on a regular basis?	☐	3
Do you have a high stress job or family environment?	☐	3
Do you avoid exercise, even stretching or yoga?	☐	3
Do you wake up more than once per night?	☐	2
Do you experience dizziness or have low blood pressure?	☐	3
Are you being treated for a serious illness, such as cancer, diabetes, or cardiovascular disease?	☐	2

Total the number of "yes" answer points (24 points maximum)

Scoring: Total the values of "yes" answer points in both quizzes.

27–41: High to Very High Fatigue Factor. Take immediate action with adherence to the Blood Type Diet, and modify the factors that are in your control.

12–26: Moderate to High Fatigue Factor. If you make some diet and lifestyle changes, you can minimize your fatigue factors. Refer to your blood type section to determine which actions you must take.

1–11: Low to Moderate Fatigue Factor. Keep it that way by adhering to the Blood Type Diet and lifestyle plan.

The Blood Type B Quiz

The following factors are known to specifically foster conditions of fatigue for Blood Type B. Check yes for each question that applies to you, then total the values of all "yes" answers.

Risk Factor	Yes	Value
Are you a non-secretor? (See page 21.)	☐	3
Do you regularly follow a low-fat diet?	☐	3
Do you regularly consume wheat or corn or their by-products (sweeteners, etc.)?	☐	3
Do you suffer from anxiety or depression?		2
Do you have a history of infection, particularly viral, urinary or reproductive tract infections?	☐	2
Do you suffer with occasional swollen extremities (ankles, etc.)?	☐	2
Do you have high blood pressure or chronic constipation?	☐	2
Are you suffering from an autoimmune disease?	☐	2
Is your total weekly exercise time under 4 hours?	☐	3

Total the number of "yes" answer points (22 points maximum)

Scoring: Total the values of "yes" answer points in both quizzes.

24–39: High to Very High Fatigue Factor. Take immediate action with adherence to the Blood Type Diet, and modify the factors that are in your control.

10–23: Moderate to High Fatigue Factor. If you make some diet and lifestyle changes, you can minimize your fatigue factors. Refer to your blood type section to determine which actions you must take.

1–9: Low to Moderate Fatigue Factor. Keep it that way by adhering to the Blood Type Diet and lifestyle plan.

The Blood Type AB Quiz

The following factors are known to specifically foster conditions of fatigue for Blood Type AB. Check yes for each question that applies to you, then total the values of all "yes" answers.

Risk Factor	Yes	Value
Are you a non-secretor? (See page 21.)	☐	3
Do you regularly follow a high-protein, high-fat diet, with little or no soy or cultured dairy?	☐	3
Do you spend more than 90% of your time in an urban environment?	☐	2
Do you regularly consume wheat or corn, or their by-products (sweeteners, etc.)?	☐	3
Do you have low blood pressure or chronic constipation?	☐	2
Do you suffer from anxiety or depression?	☐	2
Is your total weekly exercise time under 4 hours?	☐	3
Do you easily succumb to infections, colds, and flu?	☐	2
Are you being treated for a serious illness, such as cancer, diabetes, or cardiovascular disease?	☐	2

Total the number of "yes" answer points (22 points maximum)

Scoring: Total the values of "yes" answer points in both quizzes.

24–39: High to Very High Fatigue Factor. Take immediate action with adherence to the Blood Type Diet, and modify the factors that are in your control.

10–23: Moderate to High Fatigue Factor. If you make some diet and lifestyle changes, you can minimize your fatigue factors. Refer to your blood type section to determine which actions you must take.

1–9: Low to Moderate Fatigue Factor. Keep it that way by adhering to the Blood Type Diet and lifestyle plan.

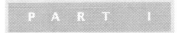

PART I

Blood Type and Fatigue: A Basic Primer

ONE

Blood Type and the Paths to Fatigue

EVERYONE GETS TIRED SOMETIMES, BUT FATIGUE IS MUCH more than that. It is not just feeling sleepy, or lethargic, or down in the dumps. Transient states of tiredness in otherwise healthy people are normal, and can usually be remedied with extra rest, dietary changes, or simply time. Feeling tired can be a normal and important response to physical exertion, emotional stress, boredom, or lack of sleep. However, when it persists it can be a sign of a more serious disorder. Fatigue that is not relieved by adequate sleep, good nutrition, or stress reduction may have a serious underlying cause.

Fatigue is an elusive concept. There is no disease called fatigue. Even chronic fatigue syndrome, which is named for its primary symptom, is not a disease *caused* by fatigue. Finding the source of the "fatigue" in chronic fatigue is like peeling an onion.

When a patient comes to my clinic complaining of fatigue, I'll ask a number of different questions to try and get at the root cause:

- Have you had a recent illness—such as the flu or other infection?
- Do you have sinus problems or allergies?
- Are you taking medications?
- Are you in a toxic environment, such as a freshly painted apartment, rooms with new rugs, high noise levels, etc.?
- Do you suffer from insomnia or other sleep disturbances?
- Have you been under extraordinary stress?
- Do you get dizzy, crave salty foods, or suffer from chronic constipation?
- Do you spend excessive amounts of time sleeping?
- Are your menstrual cycles irregular, or are you perimeno-pausal?
- Are you on a very low-calorie diet, or do you regularly skip meals?
- Are you being treated for anxiety or depression?
- Is your fatigue accompanied by flu-like symptoms, swollen glands, headaches, or joint pain?
- Is your fatigue lessened when you get extra rest?

These questions are designed to examine the underlying causes of fatigue. Fatigue may be symptomatic of many diseases. For example, it can be the result of poor blood sugar regulation, a hormonal imbalance, an allergic reaction, a fungal infection, low thyroid, an autoimmune disease, or intestinal toxicity.

Sometimes fatigue is a side effect of medications or treatments. Most chemotherapy drugs cause fatigue, as does radiation treatment. Medications used to treat arthritis, antihistamines, and some antidepressants count fatigue among their side effects.

Many autoimmune diseases, including fibromyalgia, multiple sclerosis, myasthenia gravis, sarcoidosis, rheumatoid arthritis, and lupus involve fatigue. Chronic fatigue syndrome is named for its primary symptom, fatigue.

Chronic stress, which plays a contributory role in many diseases, can also be an underlying cause of or contributor to fatigue. The repeated pressure of stress eventually leads to a state of maladaptation—

the inability to fight back. Our bodies' stress hormones depend on balance to perform their protective function. In a state of maladaptation, we are vulnerable to infections, viruses, allergies, and other attacks that continue to weaken us.

I believe that the best way to understand fatigue from a practical vantage point is to discuss its functionality—that is, how it manifests itself in a pathological state. I've isolated four distinct pathologies that are associated with fatigue. They are: immunologic chaos, stress, metabolic or environmental toxicity, and cellular blockage. These states can occur for many reasons, but the pathways often differ depending on your blood type.

The 4 Pathologies of Fatigue

1. Immunologic Chaos

Many conditions that produce fatigue are related to a breakdown in the operation of your immune system, and it is here that your blood type plays a critical role. To place the actions in context, let's look at the basic dynamics of immunity and the influence of blood type.

Your immune system can be likened to a modern army, composed of many different divisions that operate under the direction of a central command. Like the military, the immune system requires good intelligence. It must identify and attack the enemy while at the same time prevent casualties from "friendly fire." In other words, it must identify "self" (your own body) and identify and destroy "non-self" (any foreign substances in the body—parasites, viruses, etc.). Without an ability to make this distinction, your immune system could attack your own tissues by mistake or allow a dangerous organism access to vital areas of your body.

Nature has endowed our immune systems with very sophisticated methods to determine if a substance in the body is foreign or not. One method involves looking for chemical markers called antigens. Antigens are found on most living things, including the cells of our bodies. The antigen may be a foreign substance from the environment, or formed within the body. Any substance could be an antigen; the only requirement is that it be unique enough to allow the immune system an opportunity to determine if it is "self" or "non-self." Every life form, from the simplest virus to humans, has a unique antigen that forms a part of its chemical fingerprint.

When a foreign antigen enters the body, it provokes the activity of antibodies—specialized chemicals manufactured by the cells of the immune system. Antibodies attach and "tag" the foreign antigen in a manner that results in its disposal. The cells of our immune systems manufacture countless varieties of antibodies, and each is specifically designed to identify and attach to one particular foreign antigen.

Blood Type Antigens and Antibodies: So, what does this have to do with blood type? Your blood type is determined by the presence or absence of antigens. The chemical structure of blood type antigens is composed of long chains of a repeating sugar called fucose, which by itself forms the O antigen of Blood Type O. Fucose also serves as the base for the other blood types. Blood Type A is the O antigen (fucose) plus a sugar named N-acetyl galactosamine added to its end. Blood Type B is fucose plus a different sugar, D-galactosamine, at its end. Blood Type AB is fucose plus N-acetyl galactosamine and D-galactosamine. These long chains of repeating sugar are somewhat like antennae, projecting outward from the surface of our cells, on the lookout for foreign antigens.

Certain blood types produce antibodies to other blood types. This is why we can receive transfusions from some blood types but not from others. These blood type antibodies are not there to complicate transfusions, but rather to protect your body against foreign substances, such as bacteria, viruses, parasites, and some plant foods that can actually resemble foreign blood type antigens. When your immune system is attempting to identify a suspicious character, one of the first things it looks for is your blood type antigen. If it encounters one of the substances resembling a blood type opposed to yours, it creates antibodies against it. This antibody reaction is characterized by a process called agglutination (cell clumping). This means that the antibody attaches to the antigen and makes it very sticky. When cells, viruses, parasites, and bacteria are agglutinated, they stick together and "clump up," which makes the job of their disposal all the easier. It's rather like handcuffing criminals together. They become far less dangerous than when allowed to move around freely.

Agglutination is an important concept in blood type analysis. Blood type antibodies, called isohemmaglutinins, are the strongest antibodies in our immune system, and their ability to clump the blood cells of an opposing blood type is so powerful that it can be immediately observed on a glass slide with the unaided eye. This, incidentally,

Blood Type Antigens and Antibodies

BLOOD TYPE	ANTIGENS	ANTIBODIES
O	None*	You produce antibodies to Blood Types A, B, and AB. You can only receive Type O blood, but you can donate blood to all types. Because of this, Type O is often referred to as the universal donor. However, you consider all things in nature that are A-like or B-like foreign.
A	A	You produce antibodies to Blood Type B. You can receive blood from Blood Types O and A, but you consider all things in nature that are B-like foreign.
B	B	You produce antibodies to Blood Type A. You can receive blood from Blood Types O and B, but you consider all things in nature that are A-like foreign.
AB	A and B	Because both A and B antigens are present in your red blood cells, you don't carry antibodies for either. You can receive blood from Blood Types O, A, B, and AB. Because of this, Blood Type AB is often called the universal receiver.

*Type O has no "true" blood group antigen. However, it possesses an H antigen, which is hidden in all of the other blood types.

is the way a blood type is determined in the laboratory. Most other antibodies in the body require some sort of stimulation for their production, such as a vaccination or infection. The blood type antibodies are produced automatically, often appearing at birth and reaching almost adult levels by four months of age.

Most of the factors associated with your blood type relate to primary blood type, i.e., whether you're O, A, B, or AB. However, there are actually hundreds of minor subtypes, such as your Rh-positive or -negative status. For our purposes, these minor blood types don't often come into play, with one major exception: your secretor status. Although everyone carries a blood type antigen on their blood cells, some people have blood type antigens that float around freely in their body secretions. These people are called secretors, because they secrete their blood type antigens into their body fluids, such as saliva, mucus, and sperm. It's possible to find out their blood type from these other body fluids, as well as from their blood. Secretors comprise approximately 80 percent of the population.

Being a secretor or a non-secretor is independent of your ABO blood type; it is controlled by a different gene. For example, one person could be a Blood Type A secretor, another a Blood Type A non-secretor. Because secretors have more places to put their blood type antigens, they have more blood type expression in their bodies than non-secretors. As we will see, your secretor status can have a great influence on the characteristics of your immune system and is associated with many diseases.

The Compromised Immune System: In a properly functioning immune system, specialized white blood cells called B-lymphocytes and T-lymphocytes are responsible for detecting foreign antigens and producing antibodies against them. A subset of T-lymphocyte cells, called natural killer (NK) cells, is the first line of defense against infections and cancer cells. In a simplified sense, NK cells act like tiny armor-piercing pieces of Velcro cruising through your immune system. When they encounter a cell that has been invaded by a virus, bacteria, or abnormality, they attach to the cell and destroy it.

Decreased NK activity is linked to a variety of diseases, and low NK cell activity is a component of many fatigue syndromes.

According to the Centers for Disease Control, low NK cell activity is present in most chronic illnesses. In fact, low NK cell activity has even been proposed as a disease in and of itself—low natural killer syndrome. Low natural killer syndrome is characterized by lowered NK cell activity, in association with general clinical symptoms of remittent fever and fatigue persisting without explanation for more than six months. Typically, routine laboratory tests appear normal. Low levels of NK cell activity are also associated with chronic fatigue syndrome. The lower the NK cell activity, the more severe the symptoms.

Another manifestation of a compromised immune system is autoimmune disease. The word "auto" is the Greek word for "self." If a person has an autoimmune disease, the immune system mistakenly attacks self, targeting the cells, tissues, and organs of a person's own body.

Much of the damage done by autoimmune disease is the result of immune complexes, an insoluble network of antibodies bound to antigens in the bloodstream. Immune complexes form as a protective reaction to the site of injury but are harmful when they accumulate and initiate inflammation. Immune complexes, immune cells, and inflammatory molecules can block blood flow and ultimately destroy organs such as the kidney in people with systemic lupus erythematosus, or the insulin-secreting Islet of Langerhans in the pancreas in diabetics. Many autoimmune diseases, including fibromyalgia, hypothyroidism, and rheumatoid arthritis, are associated with fatigue. In fact, chronic fatigue syndrome is sometimes considered an autoimmune disease.

Blood Type–Specific Immunologic Paths to Fatigue

Blood Type O: Autoimmunity

Blood Type O is most susceptible to conditions caused by an overactive immune system. Autoimmune inflammatory diseases, such as rheumatoid arthritis and fibromyalgia, are more common in Blood Type O individuals than in those with other blood types. Inflammatory bowel

diseases, such as Crohn's disease and ulcerative colitis, also dispropor-
tionately afflict Blood Type O individuals. Blood Type O's vulnerability to a range of inflammatory problems is related to their having the
greatest levels and variety of anti–blood type antibodies.

Blood Type O's predisposition to autoimmune thyroid disease—
especially hypothyroidism (underproduction/underutilization of thyroid hormones)—is a primary factor in fatigue. Thyroid-related fatigue
is generally not significant in the morning but gradually worsens
throughout the day or starts later in the day. Thyroid malfunction may
result in fatigue of varying degrees, including a profound and persistent exhaustion. Malfunctions of the thyroid system can lead to depression, anxiety, panic attacks, and bipolar disorders because this
system affects the metabolism of the nervous system.

Blood Type O is also more prone to develop systemic fungal
conditions, such as candidiasis, and this is especially true for non-
secretors. There appears to be an association between candida and
autoimmune disease, especially hypothyroidism, and the two are often cofactors in fatigue and depression. Both hypothyroidism and candidiasis are linked to low NK cell activity.

Blood Type A: Immune System Depletion

Blood Type A is most vulnerable to immune system depletion, and one
underlying cause is low glutathione levels. Glutathione is the major
antioxidant produced inside the cells to protect them from the de-
structive effects of free radicals. In addition, glutathione recycles other
well-known antioxidants such as vitamins C and E, keeping them in
their active state. Glutathione is an essential mechanism in the immune response. It is needed for the lymphocytes to multiply in order
to develop a strong immune response, and for NK cells to destroy cells
infected with viruses or cancer cells. Blood Type A tends to have lower
NK cell activity than the other blood types, and this is in part due to
low levels of glutathione.

Blood Type B: Vulnerability to Infections

Blood Type B tends to be susceptible to viral infections, including
slow-growing viruses that produce autoimmune conditions. Type B has

the weakest defense of all the blood types against the most common influenza viruses (A H1N1 and A H3N2), and also has a tendency to develop chronic or recurrent urinary tract infections (UTIs). This is especially true of non-secretors.

Blood Type B is especially susceptible to autoimmune diseases such as rheumatoid arthritis, lupus, and scleroderma. This tendency is more pronounced in non-secretors. All types of non-secretors have genetically induced difficulties in removing immune complexes from their tissues, which increase their risk of attacking tissue that contains them. If you are a Type B non-secretor, you have an especially high risk.

Blood Type AB: Impaired NK Cell Activity

Possessing both the A and the B antigens can be compared to having two enemies standing guard at the same gate. This heightens the vulnerability to immune conditions. This is especially true when Type AB experiences impaired NK cell activity. More than the other blood types, Type AB relies on NK cells as a line of defense against infection. When lifestyle factors cause NK cell depletion, Type AB is defenseless.

Like Blood Type B, Blood Type AB has an increased susceptibility to chronic or recurrent urinary tract infections. This is especially true for non-secretors.

Non-Secretors: Heightened Immune System Vulnerabilities

In general, non-secretors are far more likely to suffer from an immune disease than secretors, especially when it is provoked by an infectious organism. Non-secretors also have genetically induced difficulties removing immune complexes from their tissues, which increase their risk of attacking tissue that contains them. In other words, non-secretors are a bit more predisposed to view their own tissue as unfriendly.

Non-secretors are dominant in virtually every immune system disorder:

- Non-secretors are more prone to generalized inflammation than secretors.
- Although non-secretors make up only about 20 percent of the population, they are significantly overrepresented

among individuals with either oral or vaginal candida infections, making up almost 50 percent of affected individuals.

- Non-secretors account for 80 percent of all fibromyalgia sufferers, irrespective of blood type.
- Non-secretors have an increased prevalence of a variety of autoimmune diseases, including ankylosing spondylitis, reactive arthritis, psoriatic arthropathy, Sjogren's syndrome, multiple sclerosis, and Grave's disease.
- Non-secretors have an extra risk for recurrent urinary tract infections, and between 55 and 60 percent of non-secretors have been found to develop renal scars even with the regular use of antibiotic treatment for UTIs.
- Non-secretors have lower NK cell activity.

2. Stress

Many forms of fatigue are at least partially caused by stress. This makes perfect sense when you realize that chronic stress can exert a powerful and often devastating effect on the body. Stress has been associated with a higher risk for many chronic illnesses, including heart disease and cancer.

The stress response is an essential part of our survival mechanism. For our ancient ancestors, stress was an intense but intermittent reality, usually resulting from encounters with dangerous predators, territorial disputes with other creatures, and the ongoing hunt for sources of food. The effective "fight or flight" instinct helped to elevate humans to the top of the food chain.

Today's stressors are usually not life-and-death battles, but they aren't intermittent, either. They're constant. It's this piling-on that makes stress so dangerous. The elevation of stress hormones that allows a powerful response by the nervous system in times of danger never has a chance to return to normal.

The nervous system has two branches with complementary functions. The sympathetic nervous system is responsible for the initial "fight or flight" response. The parasympathetic branch is responsible for relaxing the nervous system after whatever set off the alarms indicating danger has passed. The proper functioning of both systems is a critical component of good health. Together, the two branches of the nervous system communicate with your endocrine system and internal organs to help you maintain proper function and respond to a wide range of potential challenges.

For the most part, the two branches of your nervous system are antagonists. They tend to work best in balanced opposition to each other. For example, sympathetic activity causes your heart to beat faster and more forcefully, while parasympathetic activity slows down your heart rate and unclenches the arterial muscle walls, allowing freer blood flow and oxygenation of the heart muscle.

The key to the proper functioning of your nervous system is balance. Problems occur when one of the two parts of this system has a continued dominance over the other for prolonged periods of time. Chronic stress acts like a weight on a scale—it tilts the scale in favor of the sympathetic branch at the expense of the parasympathetic branch. Since many of your body's activities associated with health and healing are driven by parasympathetic activity, prolonged time intervals with the scales out of balance will inevitably lead to a breakdown.

The mechanics of a normal stress response involve the synchronized action of three endocrine glands: hypothalamus, pituitary, and adrenal. We refer to this interplay as the H-P-A Axis. Here is a simplified description of the process:

Moment of Stress

- The hypothalamus gland in the brain, often called the "master" gland, releases a messenger molecule called corticotropin-releasing hormone.
- Corticotropin-releasing hormone alerts the pituitary gland to release adrenocorticotropic hormone (ACTH).
- ACTH signals the adrenal gland to release its supply of stress hormones.

End of Stress
- The hypothalamus gland is signaled to stop producing the messenger hormone.
- Homeostasis—balance—is restored.

Normally, the checks and balances built into this feedback loop will shut down the H-P-A Axis when the stressor is removed. Unfortunately, chronic stress throws a wrench in the smooth operation of this axis and its feedback loops. The hypothalamus gland becomes less sensitive to the signal that tells it to stop producing the messenger hormone.

The critical moment in the stress response comes when the adrenal gland releases its supply of stress hormones. There are two types of stress hormones: catecholamines and cortisol. These are the hormones that are most closely linked to blood type.

There are two catecholamines released from the adrenal gland in response to stress—epinephrine, more commonly recognized as adrenaline; and norepinephrine, also called noradrenaline. When these powerful chemicals are released into your bloodstream, you experience an increase in heart rate, an increase in blood pressure, a decrease in digestive capability, an increase in arousal or alertness, and an overall shifting of your resources toward fight, flight, exercise, or some form of physical activity. The catecholamines can be thought of as the shock troops of the nervous system, acting as the immediate, short-term response to stress.

Cortisol, on the other hand, is more like an occupying army, in for the long haul. Cortisol breaks down muscle tissue and converts the proteins from the tissue into energy. The adrenal glands flood your system with cortisol in any traumatic situation. Exposure to cold, starvation, bleeding, surgery, infections, injuries, pain, and excessive amounts of exercise will be met by cortisol. Emotional and mental stress also influence the increase of this hormone.

Cortisol is essential for life; it enables us to get out of the way of danger. We would quickly die when exposed to stress if our adrenal glands stopped making this key hormone. However, cortisol is a double-edged sword. Excessive or prolonged release of cortisol disrupts the balance of a number of our internal systems. While the proper levels of cortisol will reduce inflammation, decrease our tendency to allergies, and help to heal tissue and wounds, inappropriate levels will create the opposite effect. Ulcers, high blood pressure, heart disease, muscle loss, aging of the skin, increased risk of bone fractures, and insomnia are just some of the costs of cortisol intoxication. Chronic overproduction of cortisol also severely compromises the immune system, diminishes NK cell activity, overstresses the heart, and impedes nervous system and brain function.

Blood Type–Specific Stress-Induced Paths to Fatigue

Blood Type O: Dopamine-Adrenaline Axis

In times of stress, Blood Type O tends to secrete higher levels of adrenaline and noradrenaline. This facility enables a quick and efficient response to danger. However, research shows that Blood Type O has a harder time recovering from stress, in part due to relatively low levels of the enzyme monoamine oxidase (MAO), which is responsible for, among other things, the inactivation of adrenaline and noradrenaline.

Type O's difficulty eliminating adrenaline and nonadrenaline in the aftermath of stress is also related to the activity of an enzyme called dopamine beta hydroxylase (DBH), which converts dopamine to noradrenaline. Dopamine, like serotonin and norepinephrine, is one of a series of neurochemicals involved in higher thought. Dopamine is made deep inside the brain in an area called the substantia nigra. Dopamine contributes to the feelings of bliss and regulates feelings of pain in the body. Cocaine, opiates, and alcohol produce rewarding effects, in part due to their abilities to promote the release of dopamine.

There is a "sweet spot" with regard to dopamine levels and proper thought function: Too much dopamine in the parts of the brain that regulate feelings (the limbics) and not enough in the part that regulates thought (the cortex) may produce a personality given to bouts of paranoia or avoidance of social interactions. Normal to higher levels of dopamine in the cortex allow for improved ability to concentrate, feel more relaxed, control stress, and have a more logical reaction to problems. Lower than average amounts of dopamine result in an inability to sustain attention, a tendency toward hyperactivity and temper tantrums, the ability to be easily angered, and a more emotional reaction to problems. A shortage of dopamine in the frontal lobe can also contribute to poor working memory.

There is also an interesting association between Type Os and bipolar disease, or manic-depressive disorder, verified by several independent research studies. Family studies also demonstrated a higher occurrence of genetically transmitted bipolar disease. At least two studies showed a higher incidence of unipolar, or deep, depression, in Type Os as well.

In a landmark study, investigators demonstrated that both major depressive disorder and the presence of severe life stress are independently associated with a 50 percent reduction of NK cell activity. In this study, the impact of stress and severe depression was much more important than lifestyle habits such as alcohol consumption and tobacco smoking.

Blood Type A and Blood Type B: Cortisol Axis

Blood Type A produces higher than normal levels of cortisol in conditions of stress, and has higher basal levels of cortisol at all times. That means Blood Type A always has elevated cortisol levels. Blood Type B also tends to produce higher levels of cortisol, although to a lesser degree than Blood Type A. The health costs of chronically high cortisol levels can be devastating. Sustained elevated cortisol destroys healthy muscle and bone; slows down healing and normal cell replacement; coopts biochemicals needed to make other vital hormones; impairs digestion, metabolism, and mental function; interferes with healthy endocrine function; and weakens the immune system. Adrenal dysfunction may be a factor in many related conditions, including fibromyalgia, hypothyroidism, chronic fatigue syndrome, arthritis, premature menopause, and others. It may also produce a host of other unpleasant symptoms, from acne to hair loss. There is a cortisol link to many killer diseases—cancer, hypertension, heart disease, and stroke, among others. High cortisol is often a factor in mental disorders, senility, and Alzheimer's disease.

Although Blood Type B has somewhat higher than normal levels of cortisol, there are factors that offset potential damage, including the ability to respond very quickly to stress-reducing techniques. In fact, Type B is inordinately gifted in harnessing the powers of visualization and relaxation, and therefore recovers from stress much more quickly than Type A.

Blood Type AB: NK Imbalance

Blood Type AB's vulnerability to low NK cell activity, combined with a tendency to produce higher levels of noradrenaline, makes this blood type highly sensitive to mental stress. Some research suggests that people with this combination of factors—weak immunity and high excitability—are more prone to develop cancer.

3. Metabolic or Environmental Toxicity

In my conservative estimation, at least 70 percent of all the inflammatory, digestive, or stress-related illnesses I see in my practice involve some sort of toxic imbalance. Toxicity is the underlying cause of many fatigue-related conditions.

Scientists have coined the term "xenobiotics" for foreign chemicals found in the body. It comes from *xenos*, meaning "foreign," and *bios*, meaning "life." Xenobiotics are found when the body absorbs chemicals that are not nutrients, or when normally occurring substances are modified from their natural molecular structures. The impact of xenobiotics is dependent on other factors that can minimize or exacerbate their effects. One of these factors is the influence of dietary lectins.

Lectins are proteins in foods that are capable of binding to antigens on blood cells, causing problems. The digestive impact of lectins is pervasive. They can interfere with the integrity of the digestive system, provoke inflammation, block digestive hormones, damage the intestinal lining, impair absorption, and interfere with protein digestion.

Many lectins are blood type specific, in that they show a clear preference for one kind of sugar over another and mechanically fit the antigen of one blood type or another. This blood type specificity results in their attaching to the antigen of a preferred blood type while leaving other blood type antigens completely undisturbed. At the cellular level, a common effect of lectins is to cause the sugars on the surface of one cell to cross-link with those of another, effectively causing the cells to stick together and agglutinate, perhaps their most well-known effect. Not all lectins cause agglutination; many bacteria have lectinlike receptors that they use to attach to the cells of their host. Other lectins, called mitogens, cause a proliferation of certain cells of the immune system. But, in the most basic sense, lectins make things stick to other things.

Lectins affect NK cells either directly or indirectly. Lectins are absorbed and do reach your systemic circulation. But lectins do not even have to reach your NK cells to impact them negatively. High lectin diets generate polyamines (protein breakdown products) in your digestive tract, and polyamines reduce NK cell activity. High lectin diets also disrupt your intestinal flora (the balance of good and bad bacteria in your digestive tract), and an imbalanced flora also results in decreased NK cell activity.

Blood Type–Specific Toxic Paths to Fatigue

Blood Type O: Endotoxin Proliferation

High lectin activity can have a major effect on Blood Type O's ecosystem by leaving behind undigested by-products and creating an environment where bacterial toxins, called endotoxins, flourish. Endotoxins promote the precipitation of immune complexes, initiating autoimmune reactions. Endotoxins have been known to block their own absorption. This has been termed Schartzmann's phenomenon, a poorly understood mechanism in which clearance by the liver is blocked by a small amount of endotoxin, allowing a larger amount entry into the circulation.

Blood Type A and Blood Type AB: Xenobiotics

Blood Types A and AB are friendly to foreigners, and that makes them vulnerable. They don't always recognize invaders as "non-self." In particular, Blood Types A and AB are vulnerable to hormonally active xenobiotics, which display estrogenlike activities. These xenobiotics can come from the diet, such as the phytoestrogen genestein, found in soy foods. They can also come from the environment, where they are produced as pesticides and wastes from manufacturing processes (e.g., DDT and PCBs). These hormonally active xenobiotics are of great interest to researchers; in some cases they are believed to interact with growth factors in the development of hormonal cancers, such as breast cancer. Blood Types A and AB have a high susceptibility to these cancers.

Blood Type B: Lectin Toxicity

Blood Type B is highly sensitive to the effects of certain lectins that affect mineralocorticoid activity. Mineralocorticoids are hormones (the most important being aldosterone) that regulate the balance of water electrolytes (such as sodium and potassium) in the body. Poor regulation of these hormones can cause damage to the kidneys, and may be a factor in Blood Type B's susceptibility to urinary tract infections.

Blood Type B also has a relatively high incidence of chronic fatigue syndrome, which is probably related to liver toxicity—the inability of the liver to detoxify chemicals.

4. Cellular Blockage

Your body's metabolism relies on an intricate system of intracellular communication, enabling the proper release of the energy stored from food into the cells. All organisms depend on this function. Without it, life would not exist. The power sources inside each cell are the mitochondria, which combine the food we eat with oxygen to produce energy. This energy is then stored in the form of a chemical called adenosine triphosphate (ATP).

In addition to making energy, mitochondria are also deeply involved in powering up other circuitry—making steroid hormones and manufacturing the building blocks of DNA. When the mitochondria do not function properly, the effects are as devastating as a "blackout" produced by a power plant failure. The lights go out, the engines die, and everything stops working.

For the full utilization of energy, our systems rely on molecules called second messengers, which act something like a relay team. These molecules do not enter the cells; rather, they are present at the receptor sites where they amplify the signals of the metabolic pathways, calling for the cells to release energy. A second messenger critical to energy utilization is a molecule called cyclic AMP (often shortened to cAMP), which is synthesized from ATP.

The adrenal glands, which secrete stress hormones, are intimately involved in the process of cellular energy release and regulation. Adrenaline (also known as epinephrine) triggers the production of cyclic AMP in times of stress to flood the cells with energy. Chronic stress can cause a breakdown in this cellular circuitry. For one thing, it depletes glutathione, which protects the mitochondrial engines.

This is a simplified explanation of a very complex process, but here's the bottom line: metabolic failure results in fatigue. Not a surprising result if your cells cannot efficiently harness energy.

Blood Type–Specific Cellular Paths to Fatigue

Blood Type O: Catecholamine Overstimulation
As you'll recall from our discussion of stress, Blood Type O tends to secrete higher levels of the catecholamines, noradrenaline and adrenaline, in times of stress. This allows an efficient response to danger. However, when the danger has passed, Type O has some difficulty neutralizing the hormonal activity. Poor catecholamine regulation ultimately causes a chain reaction down the line. Adrenaline continues to trigger the production of cyclic AMP, and the cells continue to be flooded with energy. The result is cellular blockage and adrenal fatigue.

Blood Type A: H-P-A Axis Breakdown
For Blood Type A, cellular blockage is most likely caused by a breakdown in the H-P-A Axis. The H-P-A Axis uses three hormones to help the body remain stable during physiological and psychological stress. The hypothalamus secretes a hormone that stimulates the pituitary gland to secrete a second hormone, which then prompts the adrenal gland to produce cortisol. When the stress has passed, the axis completes its final loop, restoring the hormones to a state of rest. Blood Type A, however, tends to overproduce cortisol and has elevated levels

even in a state of rest. This absence of *true* rest places a chronic strain on the system. Indeed, according to a recent study published in *Psychosomatic Medicine*, a breakdown in the H-P-A Axis could be a factor in chronic fatigue syndrome.

Blood Type B and Blood Type AB: Poor Nitric Oxide Regulation

In recent years, nitric oxide (NO) has emerged as an important substance capable of modifying many biological processes—including the nervous system and immune functions. Nitric oxide is a molecule with a very short life, somewhere around five seconds. It is manufactured and exhausted quickly, and because NO has a very short life span, it must be constantly synthesized. This is accomplished by the conversion of a precursor, the amino acid arginine.

NO is an important method of cross-system communication—between the nervous system and the immune system, or the cardiovascular system and the reproductive system. NO appears to function as a kind of mediator of certain types of neurons in the central nervous system. Unlike the other neurotransmitters, such as dopamine and serotonin, NO does not bind to specific sites on the nerve cell, but rather is diffused *into* the cell and works directly at the biochemic level, making it a "rapid response" neurotransmitter. NO also seems to be involved in the regulation of the opiates (endorphins) produced in the brain. In this capacity, it influences memory, learning, and alertness, in addition to its many other functions.

Although most anyone can benefit from healthy modulation of nitric oxide metabolism, there is some evidence that those individuals who possess the gene for the blood group B antigen (Blood Types B and AB) may be more at risk for health problems associated with imbalances in nitric oxide metabolism. These include nervous system disorders and autoimmune conditions such as chronic fatigue syndrome.

In the integrated human physiology, these four pathologies—immunologic chaos, stress, metabolic or/environmental toxicity, and cellular blockage—often coexist, causing a chain reaction throughout the body. Let's talk about how you fight back.

Fighting Fatigue with Blood Type Therapies

HOW DO YOU FIGHT AN ENEMY AS ELUSIVE AS FATIGUE? You begin by lightening the load on your system. In a simple sense, we are all similar to camels. Like them, we can carry a certain weight without our backs giving way and collapsing. The burdens we carry are the shared burdens of all creatures, like environmental pollution and toxins. Individually, we may carry the burdens of poor diet, stressful relationships or jobs, lack of sleep, over- or underexercise, and any number of medical conditions. If your total load is reaching its maximum capacity, and then an additional bundle—such as a stressful event—is tossed on your back, you will collapse. It literally becomes the straw that broke the camel's back. So health is often a matter of reducing the total load. That's one reason why the Blood Type Diet and related therapies are so effective. They remove a great deal of the individual burden you carry, allowing you to support the added weight of environmental burdens more easily.

The Blood Type Diet utilizes the best of naturopathic medicine, combined with individualized diet, exercise, and lifestyle strategies that support maximum health. The Blood Type Diet is nutritionally tailored to emphasize foods that support digestive, immune, and metabolic balance. It utilizes the following four keys to health.

Four Keys to Fighting Fatigue with Blood Type Strategies

1. Eat Right for Your Blood Type

Most people are aware that deficiencies in essential nutrients can make them sick. There is a direct or indirect nutritional connection to most cases of fatigue. For example, many dietary factors have been linked to NK cell activity. Failure to eat breakfast, irregular eating habits, low vegetable intake, inadequate protein, excessive wheat intake, reliance on highly processed foods, and high-fat diets all have been associated with weakened immune system defenses.

Conventional nutritional wisdom has long held the view that a healthy diet is a balanced diet. Today that view is reflected in the USDA Recommended Daily Allowances and in the Food Pyramid, which represent a uniform approach to human nutrition. However, since all humans are not alike, these standards only apply in the most general way. They address food intake without factoring in variations in the ability to digest, metabolize, and utilize nutrients and to efficiently eliminate wastes. These processes differ as people age, in conditions of chronic illness, and as a result of genetically inherited biochemical differences—such as those related to blood type.

Many foods contain components that can react directly with the blood type antigens, resulting in inflammation and the production of toxins. Other foods address susceptibilities and strengthen our bodies against these weaknesses. When we consume these, we shift the odds in our favor.

Good digestion results not only from choosing the right foods for our bodies but also by keeping our digestive systems tuned and balanced so that the interplay of all important elements, such as digestive juices and hormones, is optimized for maximum nutrient absorption and regular elimination. As my father so aptly put it, "One man's food is another man's poison."

2. Exercise to Reduce Stress

The right kind of physical activity for your blood type can help you recover from stress and resist many of its harmful effects. As a rule of thumb, there is no substitute for proper physical exercise if you wish to experience optimal health. In studies, it is clear that physical exercise significantly enhances the NK cell activities and the NK cell numbers in both males and females, and both to people new to an exercise routine and to those who regularly exercise. Exercise also seems to be the great modulator against declines in NK cell activity with aging. In a few comparison studies of immune status between physically fit elderly individuals and young, not so physically fit sedentary controls, evidence suggests that habitual physical activity can enhance NK cell activity.

The question is, what is the best exercise? That depends on your blood type. Your goal should be to reduce the overall load on your system, not to exhaust it. If you exert yourself beyond your level of tolerance, exercise can actually act as a stressor. For example, overexercise will spike cortisol levels for Blood Type A individuals, furthering exhaustion. On the other hand, Blood Type O thrives on vigorous aerobic exercise, while Blood Types B and AB fall somewhere in between.

Many factors interact to determine your tolerance for exercise—such as proper nutrition, hydration, rest, prior training, level of fitness, and the stress in other parts of your life. An important factor influencing your level of tolerance is your blood type. All physical activity, even when it is not exhaustive, usually leads to elevated blood levels of catecholamines and cortisol. However, following a period of training, most people will produce fewer stress hormones in response to exercise. In other words, once you get used to an exercise, it is not as stressful. That's what conditioning is all about.

3. Clean Out the Toxins

By balancing intestinal flora and improving digestive acid production, it is possible to restore gastrointestinal health and reduce the inflammatory responses of the system, giving it more strength to fight off the disease state. Friendly intestinal bacteria protect your cells, improve immune function, and have a positive effect on your ability to fully utilize the nutrients in the foods you eat. Blood type antigens orchestrate the proper balance of friendly bacteria in your system. Consumption of probiotics—such as lactic acid bacteria, or food cultured or fermented with these friendly microorganisms—does extend life in animal experiments and dramatically reduces a wide range of intestinal metabolites such as indoles, polyamines, cresols, nitrates/nitrites, and carcinogens that we now know are counterproductive to good health. It is even more beneficial if you consume friendly bacteria specific to your blood type, since bacteria show favoritism toward the sugars of one blood type over another.

4. Use Supplementation According to Your Blood Type

Blood type–specific supplement protocols are calibrated to add extra ammunition to your fight against fatigue. These are specially formulated for each blood type's weaknesses.

Are you ready to start? Find your blood type section, and we'll get you on the right diet for your type to fight fatigue.

PART II

Individualized Blood Type Plans

THREE

Blood Type

O

BLOOD TYPE O DIET OUTCOME: WILTED FLOWER BLOOMS

"I was diagnosed with Epstein-Barr and had debilitating pain and fatigue. I went on a very strict Type O Diet and my pain was reduced by 90 percent. I still have Epstein-Barr, but I am not nearly as toxic, so my body is able to better utilize the Chinese herbs that I'm taking. The Type O Diet gave me a huge edge and I'm finally starting to get better. I believe I will be able to defeat the virus and then withstand whatever comes my way now that I'm eating in cooperation with my body instead of against it. I've been weak and sickly all my life. After discovering that Os are the robust type, I started using my treadmill. To my surprise, I'm not a wilted flower. I'm a jock!"

BLOOD TYPE O DIET OUTCOME: A 180-DEGREE TURNAROUND

"Before I began the Blood Type Diet, I was an overweight, fatigued vegetarian. I was constantly coming down with various illnesses. I modified my eating habits according to the Type O plan. Over the past eighteen months I have had no significant illnesses. I've lost weight, I have constant energy, and I have a better sense of well-being. I have even felt a greater hormonal drive. My life has really taken a 180-degree turn since I began the diet."

Self-reported outcomes from the Blood Type Diet Web site (www.dadamo.com)

Blood Type O: The Foods

THE BLOOD TYPE O Fatigue Diet is specifically adapted to provide the maximum nutritional support to fight fatigue. A new category, **Super Beneficial,** highlights powerful disease-fighting foods for Blood Type O. The **Neutral** category has also been adjusted to de-emphasize foods that are less advantageous for you. Foods designated **Neutral: Allowed Infrequently** should be minimized or avoided entirely.

Your secretor status can influence your ability to fully digest and metabolize certain foods, so various adjustments in the values are made for non-secretors. If you do not know your secretor type, the odds are that you can safely use the "secretor" values, since the majority of the population (approximately 80 percent) are secretors. However, I urge you to get tested, since the variations are important for non-secretors who want to maximize the effectiveness of the Blood Type Diet. To find out how to get tested, visit our Web site (www. dadamo.com).

Blood Type O

TOP 10 FATIGUE-FIGHTING SUPER FOODS

1. Lean, organic, grass-fed red meat
2. Richly oiled cold-water fish
3. Olive oil
4. Walnuts
5. Seaweeds
6. Spinach, collards, kale
7. Garlic
8. Berries (blueberry, elderberry)
9. Ginger
10. Green tea

The food charts are divided into three sections. The top of the chart suggests the average portion size and quantity per week or day, according to secretor status. These recommendations do *not* apply to the category **Neutral: Allowed Infrequently;** those foods should be eaten rarely, if at all. The charts also indicate differences in frequency for some foods, based on ethnic heritage. It has been my experience that this factor has an impact upon the individual's ability to fully digest certain foods. For the purposes of blood type food choices, persons of Hispanic heritage should follow the guidelines for Caucasians, and American Native peoples should follow the guidelines for Asians.

The middle section of the chart gives the food values. The bottom section lists variants based on secretor status.

For your convenience, we have included a number of product names (Ezekiel 4:9 bread, Worcestershire sauce, etc.). However, keep in mind that commercial formulations vary among brands and regions. Even though a product may be listed as acceptable for you, always check its ingredients. Some products contain **Avoid** ingredients for your blood type. Of course, you may choose to make your own version of commercial products, such as bread and mayonnaise, using ingredients that suit your blood type. There are hundreds of delicious recipes for every blood type available on our Web site (www.dadamo.com) and in the book *Cook Right 4 Your Type: The Practical Kitchen Companion to Eat Right 4 Your Type.*

Meat/Poultry

Protein, in the form of lean, organic meat, is critical for Blood Type O, and is the key to digestive health and immune function. This is even more important for non-secretors. Meat is a good sources of creatine, which is used in the manufacture of the energy compound adenosine. A high-protein diet also enables maximum metabolic fitness for Blood Type O, increasing lean muscle mass and improving basal metabolic rate. Choose only the best quality (preferably free-range), chemical-, antibiotic-, and pesticide-free low-fat meats and poultry. Grass-fed cattle and buffalo are far superior to grain-fed.

BLOOD TYPE O: MEAT/POULTRY			
Portion: 4–6 oz (men); 2–5 oz (women and children)			
	African	Caucasian	Asian
Secretor	6–9	6–9	6–9
Non-Secretor	7–12	7–12	7–11
		Times per week	

SUPER BENEFICIAL	BENEFICIAL	NEUTRAL: Allowed Frequently	NEUTRAL: Allowed Infrequently	AVOID
Beef	Heart	Chicken		All com-
Buffalo	(calf)	Cornish		mercially
Lamb	Liver (calf)	hen		processed
	Mutton	Duck		meats
	Sweet-	Goat		Bacon/
	breads	Goose		ham/pork
	Veal	Grouse		Quail
	Venison	Guinea hen		Turtle
		Horse		
		Ostrich		
		Partridge		
		Pheasant		
		Rabbit		
		Squab		
		Squirrel		
		Turkey		

Special Variants: *Non-Secretor* BENEFICIAL: ostrich, partridge, pheasant, rabbit, squab; NEUTRAL (Allowed Frequently): lamb, liver (calf), quail, turtle.

Fish/Seafood

Fish and seafood represent a secondary source of high-quality protein for Blood Type O. In particular, richly oiled cold-water fish like cod, halibut, red snapper, and trout are SUPER BENEFICIAL for Blood Type O. These fish contain beneficial omega-3 fatty acids, such as docosahexaenoic acid (DHA) and eicosapentaenoic acid (EPA), which can help improve thyroid function, counter inflammatory conditions, and regulate metabolism. They are also good sources of creatine, which is used in the manufacture of the energy compound adenosine.

BLOOD TYPE O: FISH/SEAFOOD			
Portion: 4–6 oz (men); 2–5 oz (women and children)			
	African	Caucasian	Asian
Secretor	2–4	3–5	2–5
Non-Secretor	2–5	4–5	4–5
		Times per week	

SUPER BENEFICIAL	BENEFICIAL	NEUTRAL: Allowed Frequently	NEUTRAL: Allowed Infrequently	AVOID
Cod	Bass (all)	Anchovy	Eel	Abalone
Halibut	Perch (all)	Beluga	Flounder	Barracuda
Red snapper	Pike	Bluefish	Gray sole	Catfish
Trout (rainbow)	Shad	Bullhead	Grouper	Conch
	Sole (except gray)	Butterfish	Whitefish	Frog
	Sturgeon	Carp		Herring (pickled/ smoked)
	Swordfish	Caviar (sturgeon)		Muskellunge
	Tilefish	Chub		Octopus
	Yellowtail	Clam		Pollock
		Crab		Salmon (smoked)
		Croaker		Salmon roe
		Cusk		Squid (calamari)
		Drum		
		Haddock		
		Hake		
		Halfmoon fish		
		Harvest fish		
		Herring (fresh)		

SUPER BENEFICIAL	BENEFICIAL	NEUTRAL: Allowed Frequently	NEUTRAL: Allowed Infrequently	AVOID
		Lobster		
		Mackerel		
		Mahi-mahi		
		Monkfish		
		Mullet		
		Mussel		
		Opaleye		
		Orange roughy		
		Oyster		
		Parrot fish		
		Pickerel		
		Pompano		
		Porgy		
		Rosefish		
		Sailfish		
		Salmon		
		Sardine		
		Scallop		
		Scrod		
		Shark		
		Shrimp		
		Smelt		
		Snail (*Helix pomatia*/ escargot)		
		Sucker		
		Sunfish		
		Tilapia		
		Trout (brook/ sea)		

SUPER BENEFICIAL	BENEFICIAL	NEUTRAL: Allowed Frequently	NEUTRAL: Allowed Infrequently	AVOID
		Tuna Weakfish Whiting		

Special Variants: *Non-Secretor* BENEFICIAL: hake, herring (fresh), mackerel, sardine; NEUTRAL (Allowed Frequently): bass, catfish, halibut, red snapper, salmon roe; AVOID: anchovy, crab, mussel.

Dairy/Eggs

Most dairy foods should be avoided by Blood Type O. They are poorly digested and metabolized, resulting in indigestion, weight gain, inflammation, and fatigue. Ghee (clarified butter) is one exception because it's a good source of butyrate, which supports Blood Type O intestinal health. Eggs can be consumed in moderation. Do your best to find eggs and dairy products that are both hormone-free and organic.

BLOOD TYPE O: EGGS			
Portion: 1 egg			
	African	Caucasian	Asian
Secretor	1–4	3–6	3–4
Non-Secretor	2–5	3–6	3–4
		Times per week	

BLOOD TYPE O: MILK AND YOGURT			
Portion: 4–6 oz (men); 2–5 oz (women and children)			
	African	Caucasian	Asian
Secretor	0–1	0–3	0–2
Non-Secretor	0	0–2	0–3
		Times per week	

BLOOD TYPE O: CHEESE			
Portion: 3 oz (men); 2 oz (women and children)			
	African	Caucasian	Asian
Secretor	0–1	0–2	0–1
Non-Secretor	0	0–1	0
		Times per week	

SUPER BENEFICIAL	BENEFICIAL	NEUTRAL: Allowed Frequently	NEUTRAL: Allowed Infrequently	AVOID
	Ghee (clarified butter)	Egg (chicken/ duck)	Butter Farmer cheese Feta Goat cheese Mozzarella	American cheese Blue cheese Brie Buttermilk Camembert Casein Cheddar Colby Cottage cheese Cream cheese Edam Egg (goose/ quail) Emmenthal Gouda Gruyère Half-and-half Ice cream Jarlsberg Kefir Milk (cow/goat)

SUPER BENEFICIAL	BENEFICIAL	NEUTRAL: Allowed Frequently	NEUTRAL: Allowed Infrequently	AVOID
				Monterey Jack
				Muenster
				Neufchâtel
				Paneer
				Parmesan
				Provolone
				Quark
				Ricotta
				Sherbet
				Sour cream
				String cheese
				Swiss cheese
				Whey
				Yogurt

Special Variants: *Non-Secretor* NEUTRAL (Allowed Frequently): Egg(goose/quail); AVOID: farmer cheese, feta, goat cheese, mozzarella.

Oils

Olive oil, a monounsaturated oil, is SUPER BENEFICIAL for Blood Type O. Constituents in olive oil, such as flavonoids, squalenes, and polyphenols, act as powerful antioxidants. It should be used as the primary cooking oil. Be aware that some oils are high in omega-6 fatty acids, which can stimulate an inflammatory response. These include corn, cottonseed, peanut, and safflower oils. Secretors have a bit of an edge over non-secretors in digesting oils and probably benefit a bit more from their consumption.

BLOOD TYPE O: OILS

Portion: 1 tblsp

	African	Caucasian	Asian
Secretor	3–8	4–8	5–8
Non-Secretor	1–7	3–5	3–6
		Times per week	

SUPER BENEFICIAL	BENEFICIAL	NEUTRAL: Allowed Frequently	NEUTRAL: Allowed Infrequently	AVOID
Flax (linseed) Olive		Almond Black currant seed Borage seed Cod liver Sesame Walnut	Canola	Castor Coconut Corn Cotton- seed Evening primrose Peanut Safflower Soy Sunflower Wheat germ

Special Variants: *Non-Secretor* BENEFICIAL: almond, walnut; NEUTRAL (Allowed Frequently): coconut, flax; AVOID: borage, canola, cod liver.

Nuts and Seeds

Overall, Blood Type O should limit intake of nuts and seeds in favor of high-quality animal protein. However, raw flaxseeds are helpful for a strong immune system, providing beneficial omega-3 fatty acids. Walnuts are also SUPER BENEFICIAL. They are one of the best plant sources of omega-3 fatty acids.

BLOOD TYPE O: NUTS AND SEEDS

Portion: Whole (handful); Nut Butters (2 tblsp)

	African	Caucasian	Asian
Secretor	2–5	2–5	2–4
Non-Secretor	5–7	5–7	5–7
		Times per week	

SUPER BENEFICIAL	BENEFICIAL	NEUTRAL: Allowed Frequently	NEUTRAL: Allowed Infrequently	AVOID
Flax Walnut (black/ English)	Pumpkin seed	Almond Almond butter Almond cheese Almond milk Butternut Filbert (hazel- nut) Hickory Macadamia Pecan Pignolia (pine nut)	Safflower seed Sesame butter (tahini) Sesame seed	Beechnut Brazil nut Cashew Chestnut Litchi Peanut Peanut butter Pistachio Poppy seed Sunflower butter Sunflower seed

Special Variants: *Non-Secretor* NEUTRAL (Allowed Frequently): flax; AVOID: almond cheese, almond milk, safflower seed.

Beans and Legumes

Essentially carnivores when it comes to protein requirements, Blood Type Os should minimize consumption of beans and legumes. Given the choice, get your protein from animal foods.

BLOOD TYPE O: BEANS AND LEGUMES

Portion: 1 cup (cooked)

	African	Caucasian	Asian
Secretor	1–3	1–3	2–4
Non-Secretor	0–2	0–3	2–4
	Times per week		

SUPER BENEFICIAL	BENEFICIAL	NEUTRAL: Allowed Frequently	NEUTRAL: Allowed Infrequently	AVOID
Fava (broad) bean	Adzuki bean Bean (green/ snap/ string) Black-eyed pea Northern bean	Black bean Cannellini bean Garbanzo (chickpea) Jicama bean Lima bean Mung bean/ sprouts Pea (green/ pod/ snow) Soy bean Soy cheese Soy, tempeh Soy, tofu White bean	Soy milk	Copper bean Kidney bean Lentil (all) Navy bean Pinto bean Tamarind bean

Special Variants: *Non-Secretor* NEUTRAL (Allowed Frequently): adzuki bean, black-eyed pea, lentil (all), pinto bean; AVOID: fava (broad) bean, garbanzo (chickpea), soy (all).

Grains and Starches

Blood Type O does poorly on corn, wheat, sorghum, barley, and many of their by-products (sweeteners, etc.). In particular, the lectin in wheat produces gut inflammation and is the primary cause of celiac disease. Wheat is also a leading factor in Blood Type O's susceptibility to autoimmune thyroid disease, inflammation, and insulin resistance. The exceptions are sprouted seed breads, such as Essene and Ezekiel, usually found in the freezer section of your health-food store. Non-secretors have even greater wheat sensitivity. Non-secretors should avoid oats as well.

BLOOD TYPE O: GRAINS AND STARCHES

Portion: ½ cup dry (grains or pastas); 1 muffin; 2 slices of bread

	African	Caucasian	Asian
Secretor	1–6	1–6	1–6
Non-Secretor	0–3	0–3	0–3
		Times per week	

SUPER BENEFICIAL	BENEFICIAL	NEUTRAL: Allowed Frequently	NEUTRAL: Allowed Infrequently	AVOID
	Essene bread (manna)	Amaranth Ezekiel 4:9 bread Kamut Quinoa Spelt (whole) Spelt flour/ products Tapioca Teff 100% sprouted grain products (except Essene)	Buckwheat Millet Oat bran Oat flour Oatmeal Rice (whole) Rice (wild) Rice cake Rice flour Rice milk Rye (whole) Rye flour/ products Soba noodles (100% buck- wheat) Soy flour/ products	Barley Cornmeal Couscous Grits Popcorn Sorghum Wheat (refined/ unbleached) Wheat (semolina) Wheat (white flour) Wheat (whole) Wheat bran Wheat germ

Special Variants: *Non-Secretor* AVOID: buckwheat, oat (all), soba noodles (100% buckwheat), soy flour/products, spelt (whole), spelt flour/products, tapioca.

Vegetables

Vegetables provide a rich source of antioxidants and fiber, and the right choices can help Blood Type O balance immune functions. Fucose-containing seaweeds are SUPER BENEFICIAL in blocking lectin activity. They serve as a food source for healthy colon bacteria, thus reducing gut inflammation. Seaweeds also support thyroid function. Onions are high in quercetin, a flavonoid with potent antioxidant properties. Maitake mushrooms and green leafy vegetables promote healthy blood clotting and metabolic function. Sweet potatoes are rich in vitamins A and B_6, which stabilize immune function. Vegetables in the so-called nightshade family—white potatoes, bell peppers, eggplant, and tomatoes—should be avoided. They are pro-inflammatory and can interfere with thyroid function.

An item's value also applies to its juice, unless otherwise noted.

BLOOD TYPE O: VEGETABLES			
Portion: 1 cup, prepared (cooked or raw)			
	African	**Caucasian**	**Asian**
Secretor Super/ Beneficials	Unlimited	Unlimited	Unlimited
Secretor Neutrals	2–5	2–5	2–5
Non-Secretor Super/ Beneficials	Unlimited	Unlimited	Unlimited
Non-Secretor Neutrals	2–3	2–3	2–3
	Times per day		

SUPER BENEFICIAL	BENEFICIAL	NEUTRAL: Allowed Frequently	NEUTRAL: Allowed Infrequently	AVOID
Beet greens	Artichoke	Arugula	Brussels	Alfalfa
Broccoli	Beet	Asparagus	sprouts	sprouts
Chicory	Horseradish	Asparagus	Cabbage	Aloe
Collards	Kohlrabi	pea	Olive	Corn
Escarole	Lettuce	Bamboo	(Greek/	Cucumber
Kale	(Romaine)	shoot	green/	Leek
Mushroom	Mushroom	Beet	Spanish)	Mushroom
(maitake)	(abalone/	Bok choy	Yam	(shiitake/
Onion (all)	enoki/	Carrot		silver
Potato	oyster/	Celeriac		dollar)
(sweet)	porto-	Celery		Mustard
Seaweeds	bello/	Chili pepper		greens
Spinach	straw/	Daikon		Olive (black)
Swiss Chard	tree ear)	radish		Potato
	Okra	Eggplant		
	Parsnip	Endive		
	Pumpkin	Fennel		
	Turnip	Fiddlehead		
		fern		
		Garlic		
		Lettuce		
		(except		
		Romaine)		
		Peppers (all)		
		Poi		
		Radicchio		
		Radish/		
		sprouts		
		Rappini		
		(broccoli		
		rabe)		
		Rutabaga		
		Scallion		
		Shallot		

SUPER BENEFICIAL	BENEFICIAL	NEUTRAL: Allowed Frequently	NEUTRAL: Allowed Infrequently	AVOID
		Squash		
		Tomato		
		Water chestnut		
		Watercress		
		Zucchini		

Special Variants: *Non-Secretor* BENEFICIAL: carrot, fiddlehead fern, garlic; NEUTRAL (Allowed Frequently): lettuce (Romaine), mushroom (except shiitake), mustard greens, parsnip, potato (sweet), turnip; AVOID: Brussels sprouts, cabbage, eggplant, olive (all), poi.

Fruits and Fruit Juices

Blood Type O should consume lots of fruits rich in antioxidants, vitamins, and fiber. SUPER BENEFICIAL are blueberries, cherries, and elderberries, which lower the production of toxins. Several citrus fruits, such as kiwi and oranges, contain O-reactive lectins, so are best avoided if you are suffering from irritable bowel syndrome.

An item's value also applies to its juices, unless otherwise noted.

BLOOD TYPE O: FRUITS AND FRUIT JUICES			
Portion: 1 cup			
	African	Caucasian	Asian
Secretor	2–4	3–5	3–5
Non-Secretor	1–3	1–3	1–3
	Times per day		

SUPER BENEFICIAL	BENEFICIAL	NEUTRAL: Allowed Frequently	NEUTRAL: Allowed Infrequently	AVOID
Blueberry	Banana	Boysenberry	Apple	Asian pear
Cherry	Dandelion	Breadfruit	Apricot	Avocado
Elderberry (dark blue/ purple)	Fig (fresh/ dried)	Canang melon	Currant	Bitter melon
	Guava	Casaba melon	Date	Blackberry
	Mango	Christmas melon	Grape (all)	Cantaloupe
	Pineapple		Quince	Coconut
	Plum	Cranberry	Raisin	Honeydew
	Prune	Crenshaw melon	Star fruit (caram- bola)	Kiwi
		Dewberry	Strawberry	Orange
		Gooseberry		Plantain
		Grapefruit		Tangerine
		Kumquat		
		Lemon		
		Lime		
		Loganberry		
		Mulberry		
		Muskmelon		
		Nectarine		
		Papaya		
		Peach		
		Pear		
		Persian melon		
		Persimmon		
		Pome- granate		
		Prickly pear		
		Raspberry		
		Sago palm		

SUPER BENEFICIAL	BENEFICIAL	NEUTRAL: Allowed Frequently	NEUTRAL: Allowed Infrequently	AVOID
		Spanish melon Watermelon Youngberry		

Special Variants: *Non-Secretor* BENEFICIAL: avocado, pomegranate, prickly pear; NEUTRAL (Allowed Frequently): elderberry (dark blue/purple); AVOID: apple, apricot, date, strawberry.

Spices/Condiments/Sweeteners

Many spices have medicinal properties. Turmeric improves liver function. Garlic improves immune health and is anti-inflammatory, as is cayenne pepper. Many common food additives, such as guar gum and carrageenan, enhance the effects of lectins found in other foods and should be avoided. Use caution when using prepared condiments, as they often contain wheat.

SUPER BENEFICIAL	BENEFICIAL	NEUTRAL: Allowed Frequently	NEUTRAL: Allowed Infrequently	AVOID
Garlic Parsley Pepper (cayenne)	Carob Fenugreek Ginger Horse-radish	Agar Allspice Almond extract Anise Basil Bay leaf Bergamot Caraway Cardamom Chervil	Apple pectin Arrowroot Barley malt Chocolate Honey Ketchup Maple syrup Molasses Molasses (black-strap)	Aspartame Caper Carrageenan Cornstarch Corn syrup Dextrose Fructose Guarana Gums (acacia/ Arabic/ guar)

SUPER BENEFICIAL	BENEFICIAL	NEUTRAL: Allowed Frequently	NEUTRAL: Allowed Infrequently	AVOID
		Chili powder	Rice syrup	Juniper
		Chive	Senna	Mace
		Cilantro (coriander leaf)	Soy sauce	Maltodextrin
			Sucanat	MSG
		Cinnamon	Sugar (brown/ white)	Nutmeg
		Clove		Pepper (black/ white)
		Coriander		
		Cream of tartar		Vinegar (except apple cider)
		Cumin		Worcester- shire sauce
		Dill		
		Gelatin, plain		
		Lecithin		
		Licorice root*		
		Marjoram		
		Mayonnaise		
		Mint (all)		
		Mustard (dry)		
		Oregano		
		Paprika		
		Pepper (pepper- corn/red flakes)		
		Rosemary		
		Saffron		
		Sage		
		Savory		
		Sea salt		
		Stevia		

SUPER BENEFICIAL	BENEFICIAL	NEUTRAL: Allowed Frequently	NEUTRAL: Allowed Infrequently	AVOID
		Tamari (wheat-free)		
		Tamarind		
		Tarragon		
		Thyme		
		Vanilla		
		Vegetable glycerine		
		Vinegar (apple cider)		
		Wintergreen		
		Yeast (baker's/ brewer's)		

Special Variants: *Non-Secretor* BENEFICIAL: basil, bay leaf, licorice root*, oregano, saffron, tarragon, yeast (brewer's); NEUTRAL (Allowed Frequently): carob, MSG, nutmeg, turmeric; AVOID: agar, barley malt, cinnamon, honey, maple syrup, mayonnaise, rice syrup, sage, soy sauce, stevia, sucanat, sugar (brown/white), tamari (wheat-free), vanilla, vinegar (apple cider).

*Do not use if you have high blood pressure.

Herbal Teas

Herbal teas can provide medicinal benefits and are excellent replacements for caffeinated drinks such as coffee, cola, and black tea. SUPER BENEFICIAL herbal teas for Blood Type O include dandelion, which aids liver function; sarsaparilla, which is an anti-inflammatory and binds endotoxin; and valerian, which is an antistress remedy and sleep aid.

SUPER BENEFICIAL	BENEFICIAL	NEUTRAL: Allowed Frequently	NEUTRAL: Allowed Infrequently	AVOID
Dandelion	Chickweed	Catnip	Senna	Alfalfa
Sarsaparilla	Fenugreek	Chamomile		Aloe
Valerian	Ginger	Dong quai		Burdock
	Hops	Elder		Coltsfoot
	Linden	Ginseng		Corn silk
	Mulberry	Hawthorn		Echinacea
	Peppermint	Horehound		Gentian
	Rosehip	Licorice		Goldenseal
	Slippery elm	Mullein		Red clover
		Raspberry leaf		Rhubarb
		Skullcap		Shepherd's purse
		Spearmint		St. John's wort
		Vervain		Strawberry leaf
		White birch		Yellow dock
		White oak bark		
		Yarrow		

Special Variants: None.

Miscellaneous Beverages

Green tea should be part of every Blood Type O's health plan. It contains polyphenols, which block the production of intestinal toxins. Avoid or limit alcohol to an occasional glass of red wine. Try to eliminate coffee by slowly weaning yourself off and replacing it with green tea. The tea has less caffeine but more positive benefits.

SUPER BENEFICIAL	BENEFICIAL	NEUTRAL: Allowed Frequently	NEUTRAL: Allowed Infrequently	AVOID
Tea (green)	Seltzer Soda (club)	Wine (red)		Beer Coffee (reg/ decaf) Liquor Soda (cola/ diet/ misc.) Tea, black (reg/ decaf) Wine (white)

Special Variants: *Non-Secretor* BENEFICIAL: Wine (red).

Supplements

THE BLOOD TYPE O diet offers abundant quantities of important nutrients, such as protein and iron. It is important to get as many nutrients as possible from fresh foods and use supplements only to fill in the minor deficiencies in your diet. The following supplement protocols are designed for Blood Type O individuals who are suffering from conditions that cause fatigue.

Note: If you are being treated for a cardiovascular or related condition, consult your doctor before taking any supplements.

Blood Type O: Basic Fatigue Protocol

Use this protocol for 4–8 weeks, then discontinue for 2 weeks and restart.		
SUPPLEMENT	**ACTION**	**DOSAGE**
L-carnitine	Plays an important role in energy production. (This supplement is especially useful for Type O seniors with fatigue.)	500 mg daily
High-potency vitamin-mineral complex (preferably blood type–specific)	Nutritional support.	As directed
Coenzyme Q-10	Enhances bioenergetics of the cell.	30–60 mg daily, with food

Blood Type O: Immune System Health Maintenance

Use this protocol 4–8 weeks, then discontinue for 2 weeks and restart.		
SUPPLEMENT	**ACTION**	**DOSAGE**
Larch arabinogalactan	Promotes digestive and intestinal health.	1 tablespoon, twice daily, in juice or water
Bladderwrack (*Fucus vesiculosus*)	Supports thyroid function, blocks the activity of complement, blocks lectins, prevents candida.	100 mg, twice daily with meals
Caprylic acid	Has anti-fungal and antiseptic properties.	350 mg: 1–2 capsules, twice daily away from food

Blood Type O: Stress Management

Use this protocol 4–8 weeks, then discontinue for 2 weeks and restart.

SUPPLEMENT	ACTION	DOSAGE
Russian rhodiola (*Rhodiola rosea*)	Prevents stress-induced catecholamine activity.	250 mg, 3 times daily
L-theanine	Anti-anxiety remedy.	100–200 mg, twice daily
Valerian (*Valeriana officinalis*)—0.5% essential oils	Antistress remedy and sleep aid.	500 mg: 1–2 capsules before bed

Blood Type O: Addressing Metabolic or Environmental Toxicities

Use this protocol 4–8 weeks, then discontinue for 2 weeks and restart.

SUPPLEMENT	ACTION	DOSAGE
Sarsaparilla (*Smilax* sp)	A general tonic, acting as a digestive aid; binds endotoxins.	150 mg standardized extract: 1 capsule, twice daily
Probiotic (preferably blood type–specific)	Promotes intestinal health.	1–2 capsules, twice daily
Sprouted food complex (preferably blood type–specific) available at health-food stores or through North American Pharmacal	Enhances detoxification.	1–2 capsules, twice daily

Blood Type O: Cellular Blockage

Use this protocol 4–8 weeks, then discontinue for 2 weeks and restart.

SUPPLEMENT	ACTION	DOSAGE
NAG (n-acetyl glucosamine)	Helps bind dietary lectins, which can diminish cell metabolic activity.	250–500 mg with meals
Coleus (*Coleus forskohlii*)	Enhances intracellular energy production through interaction with cellular second messengers.	150 mg, 1 capsule, twice daily
Green tea	Improves cardio-vascular and immune health; contains xanthines, which are important facilitators of intracellular energy production.	1–3 cups daily

The Exercise Component

BLOOD TYPE O BENEFITS tremendously from brisk exercise that taxes the cardiovascular and musculoskeletal systems. Exercise is an immune strengthener, stress reducer, and a way of reducing total load on the system.

Build a balanced routine of both aerobic and strength-training activities from the following chart. If you are not accustomed to exercising or you are suffering from a chronic condition, start slowly and do as much as you can, striving to increase your time and endurance as you gain flexibility and strength.

EXERCISE	DURATION	FREQUENCY
Aerobics	40–60 minutes	3–4 x week
Weight training	30–45 minutes	3–4 x week
Running	40–45 minutes	3–4 x week
Calesthenics	30–45 minutes	3 x week
Treadmill	30 minutes	3 x week
Kickboxing	30–45 minutes	3 x week
Cycling	30 minutes	3 x week
Contact sports	60 minutes	2–3 x week
In-line/roller skating	30 minutes	2–3 x week

3 Steps to Effective Exercise

1. Warm up with stretching and flexibility moves before you start your aerobic exercise.
2. To achieve maximum cardiovascular benefits, work toward an elevated heart rate that is about 70 percent of your capacity. Once you reach the elevated rate, continue exercising to maintain that rate for twenty to thirty minutes. To calculate your maximum heart rate and performance level:
   - Subtract your age from 220.
   - Multiply the difference by .70 (or .60 if you are over age sixty). This is the high end of your performance.
   - Multiply the remainder by .50. This is the low end of your performance.
3. Finish each aerobic session with at least a five-minute cooldown of stretching and relaxation moves.

Getting Started: The First Month

IF YOU ARE NEW to the Blood Type Diet, the following guidelines will introduce you to the Blood Type O regimen over a period of one month. Follow these recommendations as closely as possible, using a notebook to record your personal experiences with the diet. In addition to factors that are measurable in laboratory tests, take the time to note changes in your energy levels, sleep patterns, digestion, and over-all well-being.

Blood Type O Fatigue-Fighting Diet Checklist

Eat small to moderate portions of high-quality, lean, organic, ☐
grass-fed meat several times a week for strength.

Include regular portions of richly oiled cold-water fish. ☐

Consume little or no dairy foods. ☐

Eliminate wheat and wheat-based products from your diet. ☐

Limit your intake of beans principally to those that are BENE- ☐
FICIAL.

Eat lots of BENEFICIAL fruits and vegetables. ☐

Avoid stimulants found in caffeine (coffee, colas, etc.). ☐

Avoid coffee, but drink green tea every day. ☐

Week 1

Blood Type Diet and Supplements

- Eliminate your most harmful AVOID foods—wheat and dairy. These foods are the primary triggers for many health problems that afflict Blood Type O.

- Include your most important BENEFICIAL foods on a regular schedule throughout the week. For example, have lean red meat 5 times, and omega-3-rich fish 3 to 4 times, with lots of BENEFICIAL vegetables and fruit.

- Incorporate at least 1 SUPER BENEFICIAL food into your daily diet. For example, eat a snack of walnuts and cherries, or add seaweed to your salad.

- If you're a coffee drinker, begin to wean yourself by cutting your daily consumption in half. Substitute green tea instead.

Exercise Regimen

- Plan to exercise at least 4 days this week, for 45 minutes each day.

  2 days: aerobic activity

  2 days: weights

- If ill health is causing fatigue, start slowly and gradually increase your duration and intensity of activity. Exercise will energize you, not exhaust you. The important factor is consistency. Just do it—as much as you're able. If allergy to grasses and weeds prevents outdoor activities such as walking and running, join an aerobics class or walk around the track at your local gym.

- Use your journal to detail the time, activity, distance, and amount of weight lifted. Note the number of repetitions for each exercise.

▪ WEEK 1 SUCCESS STRATEGY ▪
Wean Yourself from Caffeine

Many Type Os tell me they drink coffee to ward off fatigue, but this approach is counterproductive for Type Os. There is strong evidence that even moderate amounts of caffeine can activate the Type O sympathetic nervous system, resulting in a higher adrenaline release. This adrenaline release mimics hypoglycemia, even when your blood sugar levels are not actually low.

If you're a regular coffee drinker, you're probably familiar with the symptoms that occur when you don't get your daily dose. Caffeine withdrawal can cause an excruciating headache, as well as drowsiness and irritability. In extreme cases, nausea and vomiting can occur. For this reason, cold turkey may not be the best method to break your coffee habit. Here's a gentler method:

1. Begin to slowly cut your intake, at the rate of half a cup every day or two.
2. Plan ahead to substitute a healthy hot drink for your usual cup of coffee. Green tea is an excellent replacement, and it has a small amount of caffeine. You can also substitute BENEFICIAL herbal teas.
3. If you're accustomed to taking an afternoon coffee break, go for a brisk walk instead.

4. As you reduce your coffee intake, also begin to drink less coffee per cup—by making a weaker blend or adding soy milk.

5. Get plenty of rest!

Week 2

Blood Type Diet and Supplements

- Begin to eliminate the next level of AVOID foods—corn, potatoes, beans, and legumes.

- Eat at least 2 BENEFICIAL animal proteins every day, choosing from the meat, poultry, and seafood lists.

- Initially, it is best to avoid foods listed as NEUTRAL: ALLOWED INFREQUENTLY.

- Continue to incorporate SUPER BENEFICIAL foods into your daily diet.

- If you're a coffee drinker, continue to cut your coffee intake, substituting green tea.

- Manage your mealtimes to aid proper digestion. Avoid eating on the run. Make your meals relaxing, sit-down affairs. Eat slowly and chew thoroughly to encourage digestive secretions and better digestion.

Exercise Regimen

- Continue to exercise at least 4 days this week, for 45 minutes each day.

  2 days: aerobic activity

  2 days: weights

- If your work is sedentary, get in the habit of taking a couple of "movement" breaks during the day. Walk around the block, or take the stairs instead of the elevator.

■ WEEK 2 SUCCESS STRATEGY ■
Clean Up Your Internal Environment

Getting rid of toxins that inhibit metabolic activity and increase vulnerability to infection (such as *Candida albicans*) is job one for Type O. The right blend of beneficial bacteria in the gut will help eliminate the interior atmosphere that encourages fungal growth. Start with a probiotic supplement, preferably blood type specific. Your blood type antigens are prominent in your digestive tract and, if you are a secretor, they are also prominent in the mucus that lines your digestive tract. Because of this, many of the bacteria in your digestive tract use your blood type as a preferred food supply. In fact, blood group specificity is common among intestinal bacteria with almost half of strains tested showing some blood type A, B, or O specificity. For more information about blood type–specific probiotics, go to the Web site www.dadamo.com.

Week 3

Blood Type Diet and Supplements

- When you plan your meals for week 3, choose BENEFICIAL or SUPER BENEFICIAL foods to replace NEUTRAL foods whenever possible. For example, choose lean, organic beef or buffalo over chicken, or blueberries over an apple.
- Eliminate all remaining AVOID foods.
- Liberally incorporate SUPER BENEFICIAL foods into your daily diet.
- Completely wean yourself from coffee, substituting green or herbal tea.

Exercise Regimen

- Continue to exercise at least 4 days this week, for 45 minutes each day.
  2 days: aerobic activity
  2 days: weights

■ **WEEK 3 SUCCESS STRATEGY** ■
Make Time for Exercise

It's a common complaint: "My job is too demanding to fit exercise into my schedule." But with a little creativity, you can incorporate physical activity into your regular routine. Here are some tips:

- If you hold daily or weekly staff meetings, skip the conference room and do your talking while walking.
- Take the stairs instead of the elevator.
- If your flight is delayed, walk around the airport instead of sitting at the food court.
- Stay at hotels with fitness centers, and use them instead of the cocktail hour to relieve stress.

- Start a fitness club at your company, and offer rewards, such as a day off, a bonus, or a gift certificate for employees who meet their goals.
- Get involved in an industry baseball, basketball, or soccer league.
- If you drive to work, park a mile from the office and walk the rest of the way. Or get off the bus or train at an earlier stop.

Week 4

Blood Type Diet and Supplements

- Continue at the week 3 level, focusing on BENEFICIAL and SUPER BENEFICIAL foods.
- Evaluate the first 4 weeks and make adjustments.

Exercise Regimen

- Continue at the week 3 level.
- Review your progress, noting in your journal improvements in strength, flexibility, and overall energy—or not, as the case may be. Determine which exercise regimen has worked for you, including time of day, setting, and activity level.

▪ WEEK 4 SUCCESS STRATEGY ▪
Halt Your Cravings

When you crave . . .		Eat . . .
sugar	→ → →	pineapple, plum
salty foods	→ → →	nori (seaweed)
ice cream	→ → →	soy milk/berry shake
fatty foods	→ → →	banana, walnuts
sandwich	→ → →	lettuce wrap

A Final Word

IN SUMMARY, the secret to fighting fatigue with the Blood Type O Diet involves:

1. Following a low-wheat, low-corn diet that is rich in healthy, hormone-free sources of animal protein.
2. Balancing and restoring harmony to the immune system by controlling the Blood Type O tendency to interactions between the gut and the thyroid, principally manifested by low-grade Candida yeast infection.
3. Minimizing hypersensitivity to environmental toxins by improving the ability of the liver to more effectively detoxify endotoxins.
4. Improving cellular energy production and metabolism by enhancing second messenger efficacy within the cell.

FOUR

Blood Type

A

BLOOD TYPE A DIET OUTCOME: IT CHANGED MY LIFE

"I was diagnosed with chronic fatigue syndrome, and my physician prescribed the Blood Type Diet. Since beginning the diet I've had fewer and less severe 'back falls/dips' in the syndrome. If I eat 'off' my diet, I can feel it. Thanks for your great contribution for people with chronic diseases. This has changed my life!"

BLOOD TYPE A DIET OUTCOME: BETTER EVERY DAY

"For the past several years I have had an ongoing feeling of fatigue and a slight headache. The world felt overwhelming and I was always exhausted. I wasn't expecting success on the Blood Type Diet, since I have had hypoglycemia for years. I thought all of the fruit and grains would send my hypoglycemia out of control. That has not happened. I have felt stronger, and my everyday headache and fatigue have been dramatically lessened."

Self-reported outcomes from the Blood Type Diet Web site (www.dadamo.com)

Blood Type A: The Foods

THE BLOOD TYPE A Fatigue Diet is specifically adapted to provide the maximum nutritional support to fight fatigue. A new category, **Super Beneficial,** highlights powerful disease-fighting foods for Blood Type A. The **Neutral** category has also been adjusted to de-emphasize foods that are less advantageous for you. Foods designated **Neutral: Allowed Infrequently** should be minimized or avoided entirely.

Your secretor status can influence your ability to fully digest and metabolize certain foods, so various adjustments in the values are made for non-secretors. If you do not know your secretor type, the odds are that you can safely use the "secretor" values, since the majority of the population (approximately 80 percent) are secretors. However, I urge you to get tested, since the variations are important for non-secretors who want to maximize the effectiveness of the Blood Type Diet. To find out how to get tested, visit our Web site (www.dadamo.com).

The food charts are divided into three sections. The top of the chart suggests the average portion size and quantity per week or day, according to secretor status. These recommendations do *not* apply to

---

Blood Type A

TOP 10 FATIGUE-FIGHTING SUPER FOODS

1. Soy-based foods
2. Richly oiled cold-water fish (salmon, sardines)
3. Olive oil
4. Walnuts
5. Dark leafy greens (spinach, kale, Swiss chard)
6. Onion
7. Berries (blueberry, cherry, elderberry)
8. Ginger
9. Garlic
10. Green tea

the category **Neutral: Allowed Infrequently;** those foods should be eaten rarely, if at all. The charts also indicate differences in frequency for some foods, based on ethnic heritage. It has been my experience that this factor has an impact upon the individual's ability to fully digest certain foods. For the purposes of blood type food choices, persons of Hispanic heritage should follow the guidelines for Caucasians, and American Native peoples should follow the guidelines for Asians.

The middle section of the chart gives the food values. The bottom section lists variants based on secretor status.

For your convenience, we have included a number of product names (Ezekiel 4:9 bread, Worcestershire sauce, etc.). However, keep in mind that commercial formulations vary among brands and regions. Even though a product may be listed as acceptable for you, always check its ingredients. Some products contain **Avoid** ingredients for your blood type. Of course, you may choose to make your own version of commercial products, such as bread and mayonnaise, using ingredients that suit your blood type. There are hundreds of delicious recipes for every blood type available on our Web site (www.dadamo.com) and in the book *Cook Right 4 Your Type: The Practical Kitchen Companion to Eat Right 4 Your Type.*

Meat/Poultry

Blood Type A lacks some of the enzymes and stomach acids needed to effectively digest animal protein. When you overconsume meat, the undigested by-products can foster a toxic intestinal environment. For this reason, Blood Type A should derive most of its protein from non-meat sources. Non-secretors have a small advantage over secretors in the ability to digest animal protein, but should still derive most of their protein from foods other than meat. Choose only the best quality (preferably free-range), chemical-, antibiotic-, and pesticide-free low-fat meats and poultry.

BLOOD TYPE A: MEAT/POULTRY			
Portion: 4–6 oz (men); 2–5 oz (women and children)			
	African	Caucasian	Asian
Secretor	0–2	0–3	0–3
Non-Secretor	2–5	2–4	2–3
		Times per week	

SUPER BENEFICIAL	BENEFICIAL	NEUTRAL: Allowed Frequently	NEUTRAL: Allowed Infrequently	AVOID
		Chicken		All commercially processed meat
		Cornish hen		Bacon/ham/pork
		Grouse		Beef
		Guinea hen		Buffalo
		Ostrich		Duck
		Squab		Goat
		Turkey		Goose
				Heart (beef)
				Horse
				Lamb
				Liver (calf)
				Mutton
				Partridge
				Pheasant
				Quail
				Rabbit
				Squirrel
				Sweetbreads
				Turtle
				Veal
				Venison

Special Variants: *Non-Secretor* BENEFICIAL: turkey; NEUTRAL (Allowed Frequently): duck, goat, goose, lamb, mutton, partridge, pheasant, quail, rabbit, turtle.

Fish/Seafood

Fish and seafood represent a nutritious source of protein for Blood Type A. SUPER BENEFICIAL are the richly oiled cold-water fish, such as cod, mackerel, salmon, sardines, and trout. These are high in omega-3 fatty acids, such as docosahexaenoic acid (DHA) and eicosapentaenoic acid (EPA), which can help to balance immune function and reduce inflammation.

BLOOD TYPE A: FISH/SEAFOOD			
Portion: 4–6 oz (men); 2–5 oz (women and children)			
	African	Caucasian	Asian
Secretor	1–3	1–3	1–3
Non-Secretor	2–5	2–5	2–4
		Times per week	

SUPER BENEFICIAL	BENEFICIAL	NEUTRAL: Allowed Frequently	NEUTRAL: Allowed Infrequently	AVOID
Cod	Carp	Abalone		Anchovy
Mackerel	Monkfish	Bass (sea)		Barracuda
Salmon	Perch	Bullhead		Bass
Sardine	(silver/	Butterfish		(bluegill/
Trout	yellow)	Chub		striped)
(rainbow)	Pickerel	Croaker		Beluga
	Pollock	Cusk		Bluefish
	Red snapper	Drum		Catfish
	Snail (*Helix pomatia*/ escargot)	Halfmoon fish		Caviar (sturgeon)
	Trout	Mahi-mahi		Clam
	Whitefish	Mullet		Conch
	Whiting	Muskel- lunge		Crab
		Orange roughy		Crayfish
		Parrot fish		Eel
				Flounder
				Frog

SUPER BENEFICIAL	BENEFICIAL	NEUTRAL: Allowed Frequently	NEUTRAL: Allowed Infrequently	AVOID
		Perch (white)		Gray sole
		Pike		Grouper
		Pompano		Haddock
		Porgy		Hake
		Rosefish		Halibut
		Sailfish		Harvest fish
		Salmon roe		Herring (fresh/ pickled/ smoked)
		Scrod		
		Shark		Lobster
		Smelt		Mussel
		Sturgeon		Octopus
		Sucker		Opaleye
		Sunfish		Oyster
		Swordfish		Salmon (smoked)
		Tilapia		Scallop
		Trout (brook)		Scup
		Tuna		Shad
		Weakfish		Shrimp
		Yellowtail		Sole
				Squid (calamari)
				Tilefish

Special Variants: *Non-Secretor* BENEFICIAL: chub, cusk, drum, halfmoon fish, harvest fish, mullet, muskellunge, perch (white), pompano, rosefish, sailfish, sucker, swordfish, trout (brook); NEUTRAL (Allowed Frequently): anchovy, bass (bluegill), beluga, bluefish, caviar (sturgeon), flounder, frog, gray sole, grouper, haddock, hake, halibut, herring (fresh), mussel, octopus, opaleye, scallop, scup, shad, tilefish.

Dairy/Eggs

Dairy foods should mostly be avoided by Blood Type A, especially by those prone to frequent colds or excess mucus production. Exceptions are cultured dairy products and eggs, in moderation. Do your best to find eggs and dairy products that are both hormone-free and organic.

BLOOD TYPE A: EGGS			
Portion: 1 egg			
	African	Caucasian	Asian
Secretor	1–3	1–3	1–3
Non-Secretor	2–3	2–5	2–4
		Times per week	

BLOOD TYPE A: MILK AND YOGURT			
Portion: 4–6 oz (men); 2–5 oz (women and children)			
	African	Caucasian	Asian
Secretor	0–1	1–3	0–3
Non-Secretor	0–1	1–2	0–2
		Times per week	

BLOOD TYPE A: CHEESE			
Portion: 3 oz (men); 2 oz (women and children)			
	African	Caucasian	Asian
Secretor	0–2	1–3	0–2
Non-Secretor	0	0–1	0–1
		Times per week	

SUPER BENEFICIAL	BENEFICIAL	NEUTRAL: Allowed Frequently	NEUTRAL: Allowed Infrequently	AVOID
		Egg (chicken/ duck/ goose/ quail)	Feta	American cheese
		Farmer cheese	Goat cheese	Blue cheese
		Ghee (clarified butter)	Milk (goat)	Brie
		Kefir	Sour cream	Butter
		Mozzarella		Buttermilk
		Paneer		Casein
		Ricotta		Cheddar
		Yogurt		Colby
				Cottage cheese
				Cream cheese
				Edam
				Emmenthal
				Gouda
				Gruyère
				Half-and-half
				Ice cream
				Jarlsberg
				Milk (cow)
				Monterey Jack
				Muenster
				Neufchâtel
				Parmesan
				Provolone
				Sherbet
				Swiss cheese
				Whey

Special Variants: *Non-Secretor* NEUTRAL (Allowed Frequently): cottage cheese, whey; AVOID: milk (goat), sour cream.

Oils

Olive oil, a monounsaturated fat, is SUPER BENEFICIAL for Blood Type A. Constituents in olive oil, such as flavonoids, squalenes, and polyphenols, act as powerful antioxidants. It should be used as a primary cooking oil. Be aware that some oils are high in omega-6 fatty acids, which can stimulate the inflammatory response. These include corn, cottonseed, and peanut oils.

BLOOD TYPE A: OILS			
Portion: 1 tblsp			
	African	Caucasian	Asian
Secretor	5–8	5–8	5–8
Non-Secretor	3–7	3–7	3–6
		Times per week	

SUPER BENEFICIAL	BENEFICIAL	NEUTRAL: Allowed Frequently	NEUTRAL: Allowed Infrequently	AVOID
Olive	Black currant seed	Almond	Canola	Castor
	Flax (linseed)	Borage seed		Coconut
	Walnut	Cod liver		Corn
		Evening primrose		Cottonseed
		Safflower		Peanut
		Sesame		
		Soy		
		Sunflower		
		Wheat germ		

Special Variants: *Non-Secretor* BENEFICIAL: cod liver, sesame; NEUTRAL (Allowed Frequently): peanut; AVOID: safflower.

Nuts and Seeds

Nuts and seeds can serve as an important secondary source of protein for Blood Type A. Laboratory research has identified at least five natural phytochemicals in nuts that regulate the immune system and act as antioxidants. SUPER BENEFICIAL for Blood Type A are flax (linseeds) and walnuts, which are high in omega-3 fatty acids.

BLOOD TYPE A: NUTS AND SEEDS			
Portion: Whole (handful); Nut Butters (2 tblsp)			
	African	Caucasian	Asian
Secretor	4–7	4–7	4–7
Non-Secretor	5–7	5–7	5–7
			Times per week

SUPER BENEFICIAL	BENEFICIAL	NEUTRAL: Allowed Frequently	NEUTRAL: Allowed Infrequently	AVOID
Flax	Peanut	Almond	Safflower seed	Brazil nut
Walnut (black/ English)	Peanut butter	Almond butter	Sesame butter (tahini)	Cashew
	Pumpkin seed	Almond cheese	Sesame seed	Pistachio
		Almond milk		
		Beechnut		
		Butternut		
		Chestnut		
		Filbert (hazelnut)		
		Hickory nut		
		Litchi		
		Macadamia nut		

SUPER BENEFICIAL	BENEFICIAL	NEUTRAL: Allowed Frequently	NEUTRAL: Allowed Infrequently	AVOID
		Pecan		
		Pignolia (pine nut)		
		Poppy seed		
		Sunflower butter		
		Sunflower seed		

Special Variants: *Non-Secretor* AVOID: safflower seed, sunflower butter, sunflower seed.

Beans and Legumes

Blood Type A thrives on vegetable proteins found in many beans and legumes, although a few beans contain immunoreactive proteins and should be avoided. SUPER BENEFICIAL beans and legumes for Blood Type A include soy beans and their by-products. They are a good source of essential amino acids, and they contain isoflavones that can inhibit inflammation-inducing selectins from being over-expressed on the blood vessels. Soy isoflavones also inhibit the enzyme aromatase (which converts steroids to estrogens) and so help build lean muscle mass.

BLOOD TYPE A: BEANS AND LEGUMES			
Portion: 1 cup (cooked)			
	African	Caucasian	Asian
Secretor	5–7	5–7	5–7
Non-Secretor	3–5	3–5	3–5
	Times per week		

SUPER BENEFICIAL	BENEFICIAL	NEUTRAL: Allowed Frequently	NEUTRAL: Allowed Infrequently	AVOID
Soy bean Soy cheese Soy milk Soy, miso Soy, tempeh Soy, tofu	Adzuki bean Bean (green/ snap/ string) Black bean Black-eyed pea Fava (broad) bean Lentil (all) Pinto bean	Cannellini bean Jicama bean Mung bean/ sprouts Northern bean Pea (green/ pod/ snow) White bean		Copper bean Garbanzo (chickpea) Kidney bean Lima bean Navy bean Tamarind bean

Special Variants: *Non-Secretor* NEUTRAL (Allowed Frequently): adzuki bean, bean (green/snap/string), black bean, black-eyed pea, copper bean, fava (broad) bean, kidney bean, navy bean, soy bean and products.

Grains and Starches

Blood Type A benefits from a moderate consumption of grains. However, those who suffer from frequent colds and infections or have a serious illness should limit or avoid wheat and corn. This is especially important for non-secretors.

BLOOD TYPE A: GRAINS AND STARCHES			
Portion: ½ cup dry (grains or pastas); 1 muffin; 2 slices of bread			
	African	Caucasian	Asian
Secretor	7–10	7–9	7–10
Non-Secretor	5–7	5–7	5–7
		Times per week	

SUPER BENEFICIAL	BENEFICIAL	NEUTRAL: Allowed Frequently	NEUTRAL: Allowed Infrequently	AVOID
	Amaranth	Barley	Cornmeal	Teff
	Buckwheat	Kamut	Couscous	Wheat bran
	Essene bread (manna)	Quinoa	Grits	Wheat germ
	Ezekiel 4:9 bread	Rice (wild)	Millet	
	Oat bran	Rice cake	Popcorn	
	Oat flour	Rice flour/ products	Tapioca	
	Oatmeal	Rice milk	Wheat (whole)	
	Rice (whole)	Rye flour/ products		
	Rice bran	Sorghum		
	Rye (whole)	Spelt (whole)		
	Soba noodles (100% buck-wheat)	Spelt flour/ products		
	Soy flour/ products	Wheat (refined/ unbleached)		
		Wheat (semolina)		
		Wheat (white flour)		
		100% sprouted grain products (except Essene, Ezekiel)		

Special Variants: *Non-Secretor* NEUTRAL (Allowed Frequently): buckwheat, Ezekiel 4:9 bread, oat (all), soba noodles (100% buckwheat), soy flour/products, teff; AVOID: cornmeal, couscous, grits, popcorn, wheat (all).

Vegetables

Vegetables can be a first line of defense against chronic illness, providing a rich source of nutrients, including antioxidants and fiber. Blood Type A SUPER BENEFICIALS include onions, which are high in quercetin and other antioxidants that decrease oxidative stress and increase glutathione, which protects cells. Broccoli contains allyl methyl trisulfide and dithiolthiones, which increase the activity of enzymes involved in detoxification of carcinogens. Spinach, kale, and Swiss chard contain excellent antioxidants. SUPER BENEFICIALS also help detoxify xenobiotic compounds in the liver.

Tomatoes contain a lectin that reacts with the saliva and digestive juices of Blood Type A secretors, although it does not appear to react with non-secretors. Yams are typically high in the amino acid phenylalanine, which inactivates intestinal alkaline phosphatase (already quite low in Blood Type A) and should be minimized or avoided completely.

An item's value also applies to its juices, unless otherwise noted.

BLOOD TYPE A: VEGETABLES			
Portion: 1 cup, prepared (cooked or raw)			
	African	**Caucasian**	**Asian**
Secretor Super/ Beneficials	Unlimited	Unlimited	Unlimited
Secretor Neutrals	2–5	2–5	2–5
Non-Secretor Super/ Beneficials	Unlimited	Unlimited	Unlimited
Non-Secretor Neutrals	2–3	2–3	2–3
	Times per day		

SUPER BENEFICIAL	BENEFICIAL	NEUTRAL: Allowed Frequently	NEUTRAL: Allowed Infrequently	AVOID
Broccoli	Alfalfa	Arugula	Corn	Cabbage
Kale	sprouts	Asparagus	Olive	Eggplant
Onion (all)	Aloe	Asparagus	(green)	Mushroom
Spinach	Artichoke	pea	Pickle (in	(shiitake)
Swiss	Beet	Bamboo	brine)	Olive
chard	Beet greens	shoot	Squash	(black/
	Carrot	Bok choy	(all)	Greek/
	Celery	Brussels		Spanish)
	Chicory	sprouts		Peppers (all)
	Collards	Cabbage		Pickle (in
	Dandelion	(juice)*		vinegar)
	Escarole	Cauliflower		Potato
	Horseradish	Celeriac		Potato
	Kohlrabi	Cucumber		(sweet)
	Leek	Daikon		Rhubarb
	Lettuce	radish		Tomato
	(Romaine)	Endive		Yam
	Mushroom	Fennel		Yucca
	(maitake/	Fiddlehead		
	silver	fern		
	dollar)	Lettuce		
	Okra	(except		
	Parsnip	Romaine)		
	Pumpkin	Mung		
	Rappini	bean/		
	(broccoli	sprouts		
	rabe)	Mushroom		
	Turnip	(abalone/		
		enoki/		
		oyster/		
		porto-		
		bello/		
		straw/		
		tree ear)		

SUPER BENEFICIAL	BENEFICIAL	NEUTRAL: Allowed Frequently	NEUTRAL: Allowed Infrequently	AVOID
		Mustard greens		
		Oyster plant		
		Poi		
		Radicchio		
		Radish/ sprouts		
		Rutabaga		
		Scallion		
		Seaweeds		
		Shallot		
		Taro		
		Water chestnut		
		Watercress		
		Zucchini		

Special Variants: *Non-Secretor* NEUTRAL (Allowed Frequently): alfalfa sprouts, aloe, carrot, celery, eggplant, garlic, horseradish, lettuce (Romaine), mushroom (maitake/ shiitake), peppers (all), potato (sweet), rappini (broccoli rabe), taro, tomato; AVOID: agar, cabbage (juice),* mushroom (silver dollar), pickle (in brine).

*To obtain the benefits of cabbage juice, it must be consumed within one minute of juicing.

Fruits and Fruit Juices

Fruits are rich in antioxidants, especially blueberries, elderberries, cherries, and blackberries. Pineapple contains useful digestive enzymes. Lemon is an effective mucus reducer. Plums and prunes are high in the phytonutrients neochlorogenic and chlorogenic acid. These substances are classified as phenols, and their function as antioxidants has been well documented. Several fruits, such as bananas and oranges, contain Blood Type A–reactive lectins, and these should be avoided.

An item's value also applies to its juice, unless otherwise noted.

BLOOD TYPE A: FRUITS AND FRUIT JUICES

Portion: 1 cup

	African	Caucasian	Asian
Secretor	2–4	3–4	3–4
Non-Secretor	2–3	2–3	2–3
		Times per day	

SUPER BENEFICIAL	BENEFICIAL	NEUTRAL: Allowed Frequently	NEUTRAL: Allowed Infrequently	AVOID
Blackberry	Apricot	Apple	Currant	Banana
Blueberry	Boysen-	Asian pear	Date	Bitter melon
Cherry	berry	Avocado	Pomegran-	Coconut
Elderberry	Cranberry	Breadfruit	ate	Honeydew
(dark	Fig (fresh/	Canang	Quince	Mango
blue/	dried)	melon	Raisin	Orange
purple)	Grapefruit	Cantaloupe	Star fruit	Papaya
Lemon	Lime	Casaba	(caram-	Plantain
Pineapple		melon	bola)	Tangerine
Plum		Christmas	Strawberry	
Prune		melon		
		Cranberry		
		(juice)		
		Crenshaw		
		melon		
		Dewberry		
		Gooseberry		
		Grape (all)		
		Guava		
		Kiwi		
		Kumquat		
		Loganberry		
		Mulberry		
		Muskmelon		
		Nectarine		
		Peach		
		Pear		

SUPER BENEFICIAL	BENEFICIAL	NEUTRAL: Allowed Frequently	NEUTRAL: Allowed Infrequently	AVOID
		Persian melon		
		Persimmon		
		Prickly pear		
		Raspberry		
		Sago palm		
		Spanish melon		
		Watermelon		
		Youngberry		

Special Variants: *Non-Secretor* BENEFICIAL: cranberry (juice), elderberry (dark blue/purple), watermelon; NEUTRAL (Allowed Frequently): banana, coconut, lime, mango, plantain, tangerine; AVOID: cantaloupe, casaba melon.

Spices/Condiments/Sweeteners

Many spices have medicinal properties. Turmeric improves liver function. Garlic improves immune health and is anti-inflammatory. Ginger aids digestive health. Many common food additives, such as guar gum and carrageenan, enhance the effects of lectins found in other foods and should be avoided.

SUPER BENEFICIAL	BENEFICIAL	NEUTRAL: Allowed Frequently	NEUTRAL: Allowed Infrequently	AVOID
Garlic	Barley malt	Agar	Brown rice syrup	Aspartame
Ginger	Coriander seeds	Allspice	Chocolate	Capers
Turmeric	Fenugreek	Almond extract	Cornstarch	Carrageenan
	Horse-radish	Anise	Corn syrup	Chili powder
	Molasses (black-strap)	Apple pectin	Dextrose	Gelatin (except veg-sourced)
		Arrowroot	Fructose	
		Basil	Guarana	
			Honey	

SUPER BENEFICIAL	BENEFICIAL	NEUTRAL: Allowed Frequently	NEUTRAL: Allowed Infrequently	AVOID
	Mustard (dry)	Bay leaf	Maltodextrin	Gums (acacia/ Arabic/ guar)
	Parsley	Bergamot	Maple syrup	Juniper
	Soy sauce	Caraway	Rice syrup	Ketchup
	Tamari (wheat-free)	Cardamom	Senna	Mayonnaise
		Carob	Sugar (brown/ white)	MSG
		Chervil		Pepper (black/ white)
		Chive		Pepper (cayenne)
		Cilantro (coriander leaf)		Pepper (peppercorn/ red flakes)
		Cinnamon		Pickles/ relish
		Clove		Sucanat
		Cream of tartar		Vinegar (all)
		Cumin		Wintergreen
		Dill		Worcestershire sauce
		Invert sugar		
		Licorice root*		
		Mace		
		Marjoram		
		Mint (all)		
		Molasses		
		Nutmeg		
		Oregano		
		Paprika		
		Rosemary		
		Saffron		
		aprika		
		Rosemary		
		Saffron		
		Sage		
		Savory		
		Sea salt		

SUPER BENEFICIAL	BENEFICIAL	NEUTRAL: Allowed Frequently	NEUTRAL: Allowed Infrequently	AVOID
		Seaweeds		
		Stevia		
		Tamarind		
		Tarragon		
		Thyme		
		Vanilla		
		Vegetable glycerine		
		Yeast (baker's/ brewer's)		

Special Variants: *Non-Secretor* BENEFICIAL: cilantro (coriander leaf), yeast (brewer's); NEUTRAL (Allowed Frequently): barley malt, chili powder, molasses, parsley, rice syrup, soy sauce, tamari (wheat-free), turmeric, wintergreen; AVOID: agar, cornstarch, corn syrup, dextrose, invert sugar, maltodextrin, senna.

*Do not use if you have high blood pressure.

Herbal Teas

Herbal teas can provide health benefits for Blood Type A. SUPER BENEFICIAL are chamomile and holy basil, which can reduce stress; dandelion and ginger, which aid digestion; and echinacea and rosehip, which can support immune health.

SUPER BENEFICIAL	BENEFICIAL	NEUTRAL: Allowed Frequently	NEUTRAL: Allowed Infrequently	AVOID
Chamomile	Alfalfa	Chickweed	Hops	Catnip
Dandelion	Aloe	Coltsfoot	Senna	Cayenne
Echinacea	Burdock	Dong quai		Corn silk
Ginger	Fenugreek	Elderberry		Red clover
Holy basil	Gentian	Goldenseal		Rhubarb
Rosehip	Ginkgo biloba	Horehound		Yellow dock

SUPER BENEFICIAL	BENEFICIAL	NEUTRAL: Allowed Frequently	NEUTRAL: Allowed Infrequently	AVOID
	Ginseng	Licorice root*		
	Hawthorn	Linden		
	Milk thistle	Mulberry		
	Parsley	Mullein		
	Slippery elm	Peppermint		
	St. John's wort	Raspberry leaf		
	Stone root	Sage		
	Valerian	Sarsaparilla		
		Shepherd's purse		
		Skullcap		
		Spearmint		
		Strawberry leaf		
		Thyme		
		White birch		
		White oak bark		
		Yarrow		

Special Variants: *Non-Secretor* AVOID: senna.

*Avoid if you have high blood pressure.

Miscellaneous Beverages

Green tea is a SUPER BENEFICIAL beverage for Blood Type A because of its antioxidant and cardiovascular properties. Red wine contains gallic acid, trans-resveratrol, quercetin, and rutin—four phenolic compounds with potent antioxidant effects. Blood Type A individuals who are not caffeine sensitive might consider having one cup of coffee daily; it contains many enzymes also found in soy, which can help the immune system function more effectively.

SUPER BENEFICIAL	BENEFICIAL	NEUTRAL: Allowed Frequently	NEUTRAL: Allowed Infrequently	AVOID
Tea (green)	Coffee (regular) Wine (red)	Coffee (decaf) Wine (white)		Beer Liquor Seltzer Soda (club) Soda (cola/diet/ misc.) Tea, black (reg/ decaf)

Special Variants: *Non-Secretor* BENEFICIAL: wine (white); NEUTRAL (Allowed Frequently): beer, seltzer, soda (club), tea, black (reg/decaf).

Supplements

THE BLOOD TYPE A DIET offers abundant quantities of important nutrients, such as protein and iron. It is important to get as many nutrients as possible from fresh foods and use supplements only to fill in the minor deficiencies in your diet. The following supplement protocols are designed for Blood Type A individuals who are suffering from conditions that cause fatigue.

Note: If you are being treated for a medical condition, consult your doctor before taking any supplements.

Blood Type A: Basic Fatigue Protocol

Use this protocol for 4–8 weeks, then discontinue for 2 weeks and restart.

SUPPLEMENT	ACTION	DOSAGE
Methylcobalamine (active B$_{12}$)	Plays important role in homocysteine	500 mcg daily

SUPPLEMENT	ACTION	DOSAGE
	regulation, red blood cell production, and maintaining nerve integrity.	
High-potency vitamin-mineral complex (preferably blood type–specific)	Nutritional support.	As directed
High-quality "green drink"	Typically includes a wide variety of sprouted seeds and grasses with high nutritional integrity and enzymatic activity. May also contain antioxidant-rich foods.	As directed
Coenzyme Q-10	Enhances bioenergetics of the cell.	30–60 mg daily, with food

Blood Type A: Immune System Health Maintenance

Use this protocol for 4–8 weeks, then discontinue for 2 weeks and restart.

SUPPLEMENT	ACTION	DOSAGE
Milk thistle (*Silymarin*)	*Silymarin* not only prevents the depletion of glutathione induced by alcohol and other toxic chemicals, but has been shown to increase the level of glutathione.	1–2 capsules, standardized extract, twice daily. Try to take milk thistle with a meal containing eggs. Studies have shown that when milk thistle is combined with phosphatidyl choline (found in eggs), its absorption is significantly higher.

SUPPLEMENT	ACTION	DOSAGE
Selenium	Selenium is a mineral cofactor in the manufacture of glutathione peroxidase.	50–100 mcg daily
Quercetin	Promotes digestive and intestinal integrity; controls inflammation and modulates allergic activity.	200–500 mg, twice daily

Blood Type A: Stress Management

Use this protocol for 4–8 weeks, then discontinue for 2 weeks and restart.

SUPPLEMENT	ACTION	DOSAGE
Spreading hogweed (*Boerhaavia diffusa*)	*Boerhaavia diffusa* has a dramatic effect in buffering against elevation of plasma cortisol levels under stressful conditions. It also acts to reverse the depletion of adrenal cortisol associated with adrenal exhaustion.	50–100 mg daily
Phosphatidylserine	Phosphatidylserine, found in trace amounts in lecithin, is a useful supplement to help regulate the stress-induced activation of the H-P-A Axis.	200–300 mg daily
Melatonin	Antistress remedy and sleep aid.	3 mg before bed

Blood Type A: Addressing Metabolic or Environmental Toxicities

Use this protocol for 4–8 weeks, then discontinue for 2 weeks and restart.

SUPPLEMENT	ACTION	DOSAGE
Calcium D glucarate	Inhibits breakdown of beta-glucuronidase, an enzyme found in certain bacteria that reside in the gut, which blocks the elimination of toxic chemicals and hormones.	200–400 mg daily
Probiotic (preferably blood type–specific)	Promotes intestinal health.	1–2 capsules, twice daily
Green tea	Supports cardiovascular and immune system health.	1–3 cups daily
Sprouted food complex (preferably blood type–specific)	Enhances detoxification.	1–2 capsules, twice daily

Blood Type A: Cellular Blockage

Use this protocol for 4–8 weeks, then discontinue for 2 weeks and restart.

SUPPLEMENT	ACTION	DOSAGE
Siberian ginseng (*Eleutherococcus senticosus*)	Researchers believe that *Eleutherococcus* influences the feedback loop of the H-P-A Axis by reducing adrenal and thymic atrophy during times of stress.	100 mg, twice daily with meals

SUPPLEMENT	ACTION	DOSAGE
Pantethine	Deficiency of this nutrient or its precursor, pantothenic acid, results in a decrease in adrenal function with the most noted symptom being fatigue. Evidence indicates that supplementation normalizes the adrenal gland's capacity to respond to stress.	500 mg twice daily
Malic acid	Malic acid is a naturally occurring compound that plays a role in the complex process of deriving adenosine triphosphate (ATP), the energy currency that runs the body, from food.	1,000 mg daily
Green tea	Improves cardiovascular and immune health; contains xanthines, which are important facilitators of intracellular energy production.	1–3 cups daily

The Exercise Component

FOR BLOOD TYPE A, overall fitness and immune health depend on engaging in regular exercises, with an emphasis on calming exercises such as Hatha yoga and T'ai Chi, as well as light aerobic exercise such as walking.

The following comprises the ideal exercise regimen for Blood Type A:

EXERCISE	DURATION	FREQUENCY
Hatha yoga	40–50 minutes	3–4 x week
T'ai Chi	40–50 minutes	3–4 x week
Aerobics (low impact)	40–50 minutes	2–3 x week
Treadmill	30 minutes	2–3 x week
Pilates	40–50 minutes	3–4 x week
Weight training (5–10 lb free weights)	15 minutes	2–3 x week
Cycling (recumbent bike)	30 minutes	2–3 x week
Swimming	30 minutes	2–3 x week
Brisk walking	45 minutes	2–3 x week

3 Steps to Effective Exercise

1. Warm up with stretching and flexibility moves before you start your aerobic exercise.
2. To achieve maximum cardiovascular benefits, work toward an elevated heart rate that is about 70 percent of your capacity. Once you reach the elevated rate, continue exercising to maintain that rate for twenty to thirty minutes. To calculate your maximum heart rate and performance level:
   - Subtract your age from 220.
   - Multiply the difference by .70 (or .60 if you are over age sixty). This is the high end of your performance.
   - Multiply the remainder by .50. This is the low end of your performance.
3. Finish each aerobic session with at least a five-minute cooldown of stretching and relaxation moves.

Getting Started: The First Month

IF YOU ARE NEW to the Blood Type Diet, the following guidelines will introduce you to the Blood Type A regimen over a period of one month. Follow these recommendations as closely as possible, using a notebook to record your personal experiences with the diet. In addition to factors that are measurable in laboratory tests, take the time to note changes in your energy levels, allergy symptoms, sleep patterns, digestion, and overall well-being.

Blood Type A Fatigue-Fighting Diet Checklist

Avoid or limit animal proteins. ☐

Derive your primary protein from plant foods with seafood used occasionally. ☐

Seafood should be primarily richly oiled cold-water fish. ☐

Include modest amounts of cultured dairy foods in your diet, but avoid fresh milk products. ☐

Don't overdo the grains, especially wheat-derived foods. ☐

Eat lots of BENEFICIAL fruits and vegetables, especially those high in antioxidants and fiber. ☐

Drink green tea every day for extra immune system benefits. ☐

Week 1

Blood Type Diet and Supplements

- Eliminate your most harmful AVOID foods—red meat, most dairy, and negative lectin-containing nuts, beans, and seeds.

- Include your most important BENEFICIAL foods frequently throughout the week. For example, have soy-based foods 5 times, and omega-3-rich fish 3 to 4 times, with lots of BENEFICIAL vegetables and fruit.

- Incorporate at least 1 SUPER BENEFICIAL into your daily diet. For example, have a bowl of cherries as a snack, or a spinach salad with walnuts.

- If you have allergies, avoid whole-wheat products.

- Drink 2 to 3 cups of green tea every day.

Exercise Regimen

- Plan to exercise at least 4 days this week, for 45 minutes each day.

  2 days: walking or light aerobic activity

  2 days: Hatha yoga or T'ai Chi

- If you are ill or have low energy, start slowly and gradually increase your duration and intensity of activity. The important factor is consistency. Just do it—as much as you're able.

- Use your journal to detail the time, activity, distance, and amount of weight. Note the number of repetitions for each exercise.

▪ WEEK 1 SUCCESS STRATEGY ▪
Chi Breathing

Chi breathing is based upon the Taoist concept of Chi Gong, which represents energy as flowing according to certain routes in your body. Positive release is accessible through refining the breath. The calming, stress-relieving effects of this exercise are remarkable. It can be performed by anyone, regardless of age, fitness, or medical condition.

1. Stand comfortably, feet shoulder-width apart, knees slightly bent, arms at your side. Relax your neck and shoulder muscles and focus on your solar plexus (center of the body). It is okay to sway a bit—that's normal.

2. Start to rock back and forth gently. Inhale deeply as you rock forward onto the balls of your feet; exhale as you rock backward onto your heels.

3. As you inhale, lift your relaxed arms up and forward, keeping them relaxed and slightly bent. As you exhale, let your arms float down. Imagine that your hands are pulsing around an imaginary ball of energy.

4. Repeat, gradually refining the rhythm and developing the ability to "drop" your breath from the lungs to the solar plexus.

5. Repeat four to five times, then relax, letting your hands drop to your sides and closing your eyes. Concentrate on feeling relaxed and centered.

Week 2

Blood Type Diet and Supplements

- Begin to eliminate the next level of AVOID foods—grains, vegetables, and fruits that react poorly with Type A blood.

- Eat 2 to 3 BENEFICIAL proteins every day, with special emphasis on soy. Eat omega-3-rich fish at least 3 times a week.

- Continue to Incorporate SUPER BENEFICIAL foods into your daily diet.

- Choose the NEUTRAL foods listed as "Allowed Frequently" over those listed "Allowed Infrequently."

- Manage your mealtimes to aid proper digestion. Avoid eating on the run. Make your meals relaxing, sit-down affairs. Eat slowly and chew thoroughly to encourage digestive secretions.

Exercise Regimen

- Continue to exercise at least 4 days this week, for 45 minutes each day.

    2 days: walking or light aerobic activity

    2 days: Hatha yoga or T'ai Chi

- If your work is sedentary, get in the habit of taking a couple of "movement" breaks during the day. Walk around the block or up and down stairs.

▪ WEEK 2 SUCCESS STRATEGY ▪
Growing Things

Many studies confirm that sprouts made from broccoli, cabbage, Brussels sprouts, soy, kale, and similar vegetables are rich in compounds that prevent cancer and other chronic diseases. The nutritional content of sprouts is many times greater than the original food value of the seeds and beans from which they sprout. As a seed sprouts it produces large amounts of extra vitamins, antioxidants, and enzymes. The following sprouts are particularly beneficial for Blood Type A. Add to the benefits by growing your own. There are many resources on the Web and in bookstores that will teach you how.

Soy sprouts (*Glycerine max*) 200 mg
Onion sprouts (*Allium cepa*) 150 mg

Kale sprouts (*Brassica oleracea acephala*) 100 mg
Broccoli sprouts (*Brassica oleracea italica*) 75 mg
Fennel sprouts (*Foeniculum vulgare*) 75 mg
Adzuki bean sprouts (*Phaseolus angularis*) 50 mg
Alfalfa sprouts (*Medicago sativa*) 50 mg
Arabinogalactan (from *Larix occidentalis*) 50 mg
Mustard sprouts (*Brassica juncea*) 50 mg

Week 3

Blood Type Diet and Supplements

- When you plan your meals for week 3, choose BENEFICIAL foods to replace NEUTRAL foods whenever possible. For example, choose tofu over chicken, or blueberries over an apple.
- Eliminate all remaining AVOID foods.
- Liberally incorporate SUPER BENEFICIAL foods into your daily diet.
- Drink 2 to 3 cups of green tea every day.

Exercise Regimen

- Continue to exercise at least 4 days this week, for 45 minutes each day.
  2 days: walking or light aerobic activity
  2 days: Hatha yoga or T'ai Chi

■ **WEEK 3 SUCCESS STRATEGY** ■
Sleep Tight

High cortisol levels can disrupt your sleep cycle. You may have to work harder to stay energized. Try to establish a regular sleep schedule and adhere to it as closely as possible. When you have a normal sleep-wake rhythm, it reduces cortisol levels. During the day, schedule at least two breaks of twenty minutes each for complete relaxation. Combat sleep disturbances with regular exercise and a relaxing pre-bedtime routine. A light snack before bedtime will help raise your blood sugar levels and improve sleep. If these strategies don't work, ask your doctor about the following supplement:

Methylcobalamin (active vitamin B$_{12}$): 1 to 3 mg per day taken in the morning. This vitamin enables deep sleep, and helps you wake feeling more rested. Methylcobalamin also helps folic acid lower homocysteine.

Week 4

Blood Type Diet and Supplements

- Continue at the week 3 level, focusing on BENEFICIAL and SUPER BENEFICIAL foods.

Exercise Regimen

- Continue at the week 3 level.
- Review your progress, noting in your journal improvements in strength and flexibility. Determine which exercise regimen has worked for you, including time of day, setting, and activity level.

▪ WEEK 4 SUCCESS STRATEGY ▪
Maximize Energy with the Right Eating Schedule

For Blood Type A, the timing of your meals can be almost as important as what you eat. This is particularly true if you're trying to lose weight. The following are helpful guidelines:

- Never skip meals. You won't be "saving" calories, as the metabolic reaction will foil your efforts.
- Make breakfast your most important protein-rich meal of the day. The result will be an efficient metabolism all day long.
- Eat on a sliding scale: big breakfast, medium lunch, small dinner.
- Resist the late-night munchies, but if you have problems regulating blood sugar, have a small protein snack—yogurt or soy milk—before bedtime.

A Final Word

IN SUMMARY, the secret to fighting fatigue with the Blood Type A Diet involves:

1. Maximizing overall health by eating a diet rich in soy protein, BENEFICIAL seafood, and green vegetables.
2. Minimizing the consumption of toxic lectins abundant in certain grains, beans, and vegetables that are not right for your type.
3. Improving metabolic health, lowering cholesterol, and reducing cardiovascular disease risk by avoiding red meat and high-fat foods.
4. Reducing stress and improving fitness by engaging in regular exercise appropriate for your blood type.
5. Using supplements to improve digestive health, reduce stress, and build immunity against disease.

F I V E

Blood Type

BLOOD TYPE B DIET OUTCOME: WONDER WOMAN
"I've followed the Blood Type B Diet for more than a year now. Principally, I've eliminated chicken, corn products, and most legumes from my diet. The most exciting result is an improvement in my immunity. I haven't had a cold or even a sniffle since I started the diet. In the past, I would have had at least three serious colds in this length of time. I've begun to feel like Wonder Woman when it comes to fending off the little bugs that go around. I've experienced a tremendous upsurge in energy and sense of well-being. I didn't realize until I started getting enough protein, how protein-deprived I must have been from years of avoiding meat. I credit the Blood Type Diet with an overall change in my body chemistry that has allowed me to moderate my disordered eating and slowly begin to lose weight."

BLOOD TYPE B DIET OUTCOME: GROWING ENERGY
"Last spring my herb and vegetable gardens were a burden to me. I had to push myself to go outside and work. This spring I'm eager to get out there. It's still very hard, tiring work, but I recover much more quickly than I used to, and, although I get hungry, I don't get the hypoglycemic shakes anymore."

Self-reported outcomes from the Blood Type Diet Web site (www.dadamo.com)

Blood Type B: The Foods

THE BLOOD TYPE B Fatigue Diet is specifically adapted to provide the maximum nutritional support to fight fatigue. A new category, **Super Beneficial,** highlights powerful disease-fighting foods for Blood Type B. The **Neutral** category has also been adjusted to de-emphasize foods that are less advantageous for you. Foods designated **Neutral: Allowed Infrequently** should be minimized or avoided entirely.

Your secretor status can influence your ability to fully digest and metabolize certain foods, so various adjustments in the values are made for non-secretors. If you do not know your secretor type, the odds are that you can safely use the "secretor" values, since the majority of the population (approximately 80 percent) are secretors. However, I urge you to get tested, since the variations are important for non-secretors who want to maximize the effectiveness of the Blood Type Diet. To find out how to get tested, visit our Web site (www. dadamo.com).

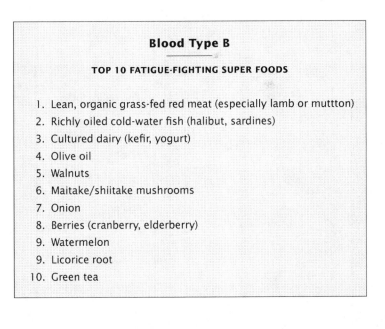

Blood Type B

TOP 10 FATIGUE-FIGHTING SUPER FOODS

1. Lean, organic grass-fed red meat (especially lamb or muttton)
2. Richly oiled cold-water fish (halibut, sardines)
3. Cultured dairy (kefir, yogurt)
4. Olive oil
5. Walnuts
6. Maitake/shiitake mushrooms
7. Onion
8. Berries (cranberry, elderberry)
9. Watermelon
9. Licorice root
10. Green tea

The food charts are divided into three sections. The top of the chart suggests the average portion size and quantity per week or day, according to secretor status. These recommendations do *not* apply to the category **Neutral: Allowed Infrequently;** those foods should be eaten rarely, if at all. The charts also indicate differences in frequency for some foods based on ethnic heritage. It has been my experience that this factor has an impact upon the individual's ability to fully digest certain foods. For the purposes of blood type food choices, persons of Hispanic heritage should follow the guidelines for Caucasians, and American Native peoples should follow the guidelines for Asians.

The middle section of the chart gives the food values. The bottom section lists variants based on secretor status.

For your convenience, we have included a number of product names (Ezekiel 4:9 bread, Worcestershire sauce, etc.). However, keep in mind that commercial formulations vary among brands and regions. Even though a product may be listed as acceptable for you, always check its ingredients. Some products contain **Avoid** ingredients for your blood type. Of course, you may choose to make your own version of commercial products, such as bread and mayonnaise, using ingredients that suit your blood type. There are hundreds of delicious recipes for every blood type available on our Web site (www.dadamo.com) and in the book *Cook Right 4 Your Type: The Practical Kitchen Companion to Eat Right 4 Your Type.*

Meat/Poultry

Blood Type B is able to efficiently metabolize animal protein, but there are limitations that require careful dietary navigation. Chicken, one of the most popular food choices, disagrees with Blood Type B, because of a B-specific agglutinin called a galectin, contained in the organ and muscle meat. This galectin can trigger inflammatory and autoimmune conditions. Turkey does not contain this lectin and can be eaten as an excellent alternative to chicken. Choose only the best quality (preferably free-range), chemical-, antibiotic-, and pesticide-free low-fat meats and poultry. Grass-fed cattle are far superior to grain-fed.

BLOOD TYPE B: MEATS/POULTRY

Portion: 4–6 oz (men); 2–5 oz (women and children)

	African	Caucasian	Asian
Secretor	3–6	2–6	2–5
Non-Secretor	4–7	4–7	4–7
		Times per week	

SUPER BENEFICIAL	BENEFICIAL	NEUTRAL: Allowed Frequently	NEUTRAL: Allowed Infrequently	AVOID
Goat	Rabbit	Beef		All commercially processed meats
Lamb	Venison	Buffalo		Bacon/ham/pork
Mutton		Liver (calf)		Chicken
		Ostrich		Cornish hen
		Pheasant		Duck
		Turkey		Goose
		Veal		Grouse
				Guinea hen
				Heart (beef)
				Horse
				Partridge
				Quail
				Squab
				Squirrel
				Sweetbreads
				Turtle

Special Variants: *Non-Secretor* BENEFICIAL: liver (calf); NEUTRAL (Allowed Frequently): heart (beef), horse, squab, sweetbreads.

Fish/Seafood

Richly oiled cold-water fish, such as halibut, mackerel, cod, salmon, and sardines, are especially good protein sources for Type B, since they are excellent sources of omega-3 fatty acids. Avoid shellfish, which can trigger allergic reactions. Salmon, halibut, and sardines are good sources of phosphorus (needed for energy production): ATP (adenosine triphosphate) and ADP (adenosine diphosphate).

BLOOD TYPE B: FISH/SEAFOOD			
Portion: 4–6 oz (men); 2–5 oz (women and children)			
	African	Caucasian	Asian
Secretor	4–5	3–5	3–5
Non-Secretor	4–5	4–5	4–5
		Times per week	

SUPER BENEFICIAL	BENEFICIAL	NEUTRAL: Allowed Frequently	NEUTRAL: Allowed Infrequently	AVOID
Cod	Caviar	Abalone	Herring	Anchovy
Halibut	(sturgeon)	Bluefish	(pickled/	Barracuda
Mackerel	Croaker	Bullhead	smoked)	Bass (all)
Sardine	Flounder	Carp	Salmon	Beluga
	Grouper	Catfish	(smoked)	Butterfish
	Haddock	Chub	Scallop	Clam
	Hake	Cusk		Conch
	Harvest	Drum		Crab
	fish	Halfmoon		Crayfish
	Mahi-mahi	fish		Eel
	Monkfish	Herring		Frog
	Perch	(fresh)		Lobster
	(ocean)	Mullet		Mussel
	Pickerel	Muskel-		Octopus
	Pike	lunge		Oyster
	Porgy	Opaleye		Pollock
	Salmon			Shrimp

SUPER BENEFICIAL	BENEFICIAL	NEUTRAL: Allowed Frequently	NEUTRAL: Allowed Infrequently	AVOID
	Shad	Orange roughy		Snail (*Helix pomatia/ escargot*)
	Sole	Parrot fish		Trout (all)
	Sturgeon	Perch (silver/ white/ yellow)		Yellowtail
		Pompano		
		Red snapper		
		Rosefish		
		Scrod		
		Scup		
		Shark		
		Smelt		
		Sole (gray)		
		Squid (calamari)		
		Sucker		
		Sunfish		
		Swordfish		
		Tilapia		
		Tilefish		
		Tuna		
		Weakfish		
		Whitefish		
		Whiting		

Special Variants: *Non-Secretor* BENEFICIAL: carp; NEUTRAL (Allowed Frequently): barracuda, butterfish, caviar (sturgeon), flounder, halibut, pike, salmon, sole (gray), snail (*Helix pomatia*/escargot), yellowtail; AVOID: scallop.

Dairy/Eggs

Dairy products, especially cultured dairy products, can be eaten by almost all Blood Type B secretors, and to a lesser degree by non-secretors. Cultured dairy, such as yogurt and kefir, is particularly good for Blood Type B; these foods help build a healthy intestinal environment. Ghee (clarified butter) contains BENEFICIAL fatty acids believed to promote intestinal balance. Non-secretors should be wary of eating too much cheese, as they are more sensitive to many of the microbial strains in aged cheeses. This sensitivity is greater for those of African ancestry, but the sensitivity can also be found in Caucasian and Asian populations. Cheese consumption should also be limited for those who suffer from recurrent infections or allergies, as cheese can trigger inflammation and produce excess mucus. Eggs and some dairy products are good sources of phosphorus (needed for energy production: ATP (adenosine triphosphate) and ADP (adenosine diphosphate). Do your best to find dairy products that are both hormone-free and organic.

BLOOD TYPE B: EGGS			
Portion: 1 egg			
	African	Caucasian	Asian
Secretor	3–4	3–4	3–5
Non-Secretor	5–6	5–6	5–6
		Times per week	

BLOOD TYPE B: MILK AND YOGURT			
Portion: 4–6 oz (men); 2–5 oz (women and children)			
	African	Caucasian	Asian
Secretor	3–5	3–4	3–4
Non-Secretor	1–3	2–4	1–3
		Times per week	

BLOOD TYPE B: CHEESE

Portion: 3 oz (men); 2 oz (women and children)

	African	Caucasian	Asian
Secretor	3–4	3–5	3–4
Non-Secretor	1–4	1–4	1–4
		Times per week	

SUPER BENEFICIAL	BENEFICIAL	NEUTRAL: Allowed Frequently	NEUTRAL: Allowed Infrequently	AVOID
Ghee (clarified butter)	Cottage cheese	Camembert	Brie	American cheese
Kefir	Farmer cheese	Casein	Butter	Blue cheese
Yogurt	Feta	Cream cheese	Buttermilk	Egg (duck/ goose/ quail)
	Goat cheese	Edam	Cheddar	Ice cream
	Milk (cow/ goat)	Egg (chicken)	Colby	
	Mozzarella	Emmenthal	Half-and- half	
	Paneer	Gouda	Jarlsberg	
	Ricotta	Gruyère	Monterey Jack	
		Neufchâtel	Muenster	
		Parmesan	Sherbet	
		Provolone	Swiss cheese	
		Quark	Whey	
		Sour cream		

Special Variants: *Non-Secretor* BENEFICIAL: whey; NEUTRAL (Allowed Frequently): cottage cheese, milk (cow); AVOID: Camembert, cheddar, Emmenthal, Jarlsberg, Monterey Jack, Muenster, Parmesan, provolone, Swiss cheese.

Oils

Blood Type B does best on monounsaturated oils and oils rich in omega series fatty acids. Olive oil fits the bill in both regards. Constituents in olive oil, such as flavonoids, squalenes, and polyphenols, act as powerful antioxidants. It should be used as the primary cooking oil.

Sesame, sunflower, and corn oils should be avoided as they contain immunoreactive proteins that impair Blood Type B digestion.

BLOOD TYPE B: OILS			
Portion: 1 tblsp			
	African	Caucasian	Asian
Secretor	5–8	5–8	5–8
Non-Secretor	3–5	3–7	3–6
			Times per week

SUPER BENEFICIAL	BENEFICIAL	NEUTRAL: Allowed Frequently	NEUTRAL: Allowed Infrequently	AVOID
Olive	Flax (linseed)	Almond Black currant seed Cod liver Evening primrose Walnut	Wheat germ	Avocado Canola Castor Coconut Corn Cottonseed Peanut Safflower Sesame Soy Sunflower

Special Variants: *Non-Secretor* BENEFICIAL: black currant seed, walnut.

Nuts and Seeds

Nuts and seeds can be an important secondary source of protein for Blood Type B. Walnuts are highly effective in inhibiting gastrointestinal toxicity; flax (linseeds) contain BENEFICIAL immunity-enhancing chemicals. As with other aspects of the Blood Type B Diet Plan, there are some idiosyncratic elements to the choice of seeds and nuts: Several, such as sunflower and sesame, have B-agglutinating lectins and should be avoided.

BLOOD TYPE B: NUTS AND SEEDS

Portion: Whole (handful); Nut Butters (2 tblsp)

	African	Caucasian	Asian
Secretor	4–7	4–7	4–7
Non-Secretor	5–7	5–7	5–7
	Times per week		

SUPER BENEFICIAL	BENEFICIAL	NEUTRAL: Allowed Frequently	NEUTRAL: Allowed Infrequently	AVOID
Flax		Almond	Litchi	Cashew
Walnut (black)		Almond butter	Macadamia	Filbert (hazelnut)
		Beechnut	Pecan	Peanut
		Brazil nut		Peanut butter
		Butternut		Pignolia (pine nut)
		Chestnut		Pistachio
		Hickory		Poppy seed
		Walnut (English)		Pumpkin seed
				Safflower seed
				Sesame butter (tahini)
				Sesame seed
				Sunflower seed

Special Variants: *Non-Secretor* BENEFICIAL: walnut (English); NEUTRAL (Allowed Frequently): pumpkin seed.

Beans and Legumes

Blood Type B can do well on the proteins found in many beans and legumes, although this food category does contain more than a few beans with problematic lectins. Soy products should be de-emphasized, as they are rich in a class of enzymes that can interact negatively with the B antigen. Several beans, such as mung beans, contain B-agglutinating lectins and should be avoided.

BLOOD TYPE B: OILS			
Portion: 1 cup (cooked)			
	African	Caucasian	Asian
Secretor	5–7	5–7	5–7
Non-Secretor	3–5	3–5	3–5
		Times per week	

SUPER BENEFICIAL	BENEFICIAL	NEUTRAL: Allowed Frequently	NEUTRAL: Allowed Infrequently	AVOID
	Bean (green/ snap/ string)	Cannellini bean	Soy bean	Adzuki bean
		Copper bean		Black bean
	Fava (broad) bean	Jicama bean		Black-eyed pea
	Kidney bean	Pea (green/ pod/ snow)		Garbanzo (chickpea)
	Lima bean			Lentil (all)
	Navy bean	Tamarind bean		Mung bean/ sprout
	Northern bean	White bean		Pinto bean
				Soy cheese
				Soy milk
				Soy, miso
				Soy, tempeh
				Soy, tofu

Special Variants: *Non-Secretor* NEUTRAL (Allowed Frequently): bean (green/snap/ string), fava (broad) bean, kidney bean, lima bean, navy bean, northern bean, soy milk; AVOID: soy bean.

Grains and Starches

Grains are a leading factor in triggering inflammatory and autoimmune conditions in Blood Type B. The wheat agglutinin is particularly harmful, as is the lectin in corn. Non-secretors have an even greater sensitivity. Sprouted grains, such as Essene bread (manna), are the exception. Sprouting makes the grains less reactive to the Type B immune system.

BLOOD TYPE B: GRAINS AND STARCHES			
Portion: ½ cup dry (grains or pastas); 1 muffin; 2 slices of bread			
	African	Caucasian	Asian
Secretor	5–7	5–9	5–9
Non-Secretor	3–5	3–5	3–5
		Times per week	

SUPER BENEFICIAL	BENEFICIAL	NEUTRAL: Allowed Frequently	NEUTRAL: Allowed Infrequently	AVOID
	Essene bread (manna)	Barley	Rice flour	Amaranth
	Ezekiel 4:9 bread	Quinoa	Soy flour/ products	Buckwheat
	Millet	Spelt flour/ products	Wheat (refined/ unbleached)	Cornmeal
	Oat bran		Wheat (semolina)	Couscous
	Oat flour		Wheat (white flour)	Grits
	Oatmeal			Kamut
	Rice bran			Popcorn
	Rice cake			Rice (wild)
	Rice milk			Rye
	Spelt (whole)			Rye flour
				Soba noodles (100% buckwheat)
				Sorghum
				Tapioca

SUPER BENEFICIAL	BENEFICIAL	NEUTRAL: Allowed Frequently	NEUTRAL: Allowed Infrequently	AVOID
				Teff
				Wheat (whole)
				Wheat bran
				Wheat germ

Special Variants: *Non-Secretor* NEUTRAL (Allowed Frequently): amaranth, Ezekiel 4:9 bread, oat (all), rice (wild), sorghum, spelt (whole), tapioca; AVOID: soy flour/products, wheat (all).

Vegetables

Vegetables can be your first line of defense against chronic disease. They provide a rich source of antioxidants and fiber and are essential to intestinal health. SUPER BENEFICIAL vegetables, such as maitake and shiitake mushrooms, are rich sources of antioxidants and immune modulators. Cabbage, cauliflower, and Brussels sprouts reduce the production of polyamines in the digestive tract. Onions and broccoli are potent detoxifiers. Broccoli contains allyl methyl trisulfide and dithiolthiones, which increase the activity of enzymes involved in detoxification.

Tomatoes contain a lectin that reacts with the saliva and digestive juices of Blood Type B secretors, although it does not appear to react with non-secretors. Corn has B-agglutinating activity and should be avoided.

An item's value also applies to its juice, unless otherwise noted.

BLOOD TYPE B: VEGETABLES

Portion: 1 cup, prepared (cooked or raw)

	African	Caucasian	Asian
Secretor Super/ Beneficials	Unlimited	Unlimited	Unlimited
Secretor Neutrals	2–5	2–5	2–5
Non-Secretor Super/ Beneficials	Unlimited	Unlimited	Unlimited
Non-Secretor Neutrals	2–3	2–3	2–3
	Times per day		

SUPER BENEFICIAL	BENEFICIAL	NEUTRAL: Allowed Frequently	NEUTRAL: Allowed Infrequently	AVOID
Broccoli	Beet	Alfalfa	Potato	Aloe
Brussels sprouts	Beet greens	sprouts		Artichoke
Cabbage	Carrot	Arugula		Corn
Cabbage (juice)*	Collards	Asparagus		Olive (all)
Cauliflower	Eggplant	Asparagus pea		Pumpkin
Mushroom (maitake/ shiitake)	Kale	Bamboo shoots		Radish/ sprouts
Onion (all)	Mustard greens	Bok choy		Rhubarb
	Parsnip	Carrot (juice)		Tomato
	Peppers (all)	Celeriac		
	Potato (sweet)	Celery		
	Yam	Chicory		
		Cucumber		
		Daikon radish		
		Dandelion		
		Endive		
		Escarole		
		Fennel		
		Fiddlehead fern		
		Horse- radish		
		Kohlrabi		
		Leek		
		Lettuce (all)		

SUPER BENEFICIAL	BENEFICIAL	NEUTRAL: Allowed Frequently	NEUTRAL: Allowed Infrequently	AVOID
		Mushroom (abalone/ enoki/ oyster/ porto- bello/ silver dollar/ straw/ tree ear)		
		Okra		
		Oyster plant		
		Pickle (in brine or vinegar)		
		Poi		
		Radicchio		
		Rappini (broccoli rabe)		
		Rutabaga		
		Scallion		
		Seaweeds		
		Shallot		
		Spinach		
		Squash (all)		
		Swiss chard		
		Taro		
		Turnip		
		Water chestnut		

SUPER BENEFICIAL	BENEFICIAL	NEUTRAL: Allowed Frequently	NEUTRAL: Allowed Infrequently	AVOID
		Watercress		
		Yucca		
		Zucchini		

Special Variants: *Non-Secretor* BENEFICIAL: okra; NEUTRAL (Allowed Frequently): artichoke, cabbage, eggplant, peppers (all), pumpkin, tomato; AVOID: potato.

*To obtain the benefits of cabbage juice, it must be consumed within one minute of juicing.

Fruits and Fruit Juices

Many SUPER BENEFICIAL fruits have powerful antioxidant effects that help to reduce infection. Elderberries are particularly effective against viral infections. Watermelon improves nitric oxide synthesis and reduces edema. Plums are high in the phytonutrients neochlorogenic and chlorogenic acids. These substances are classified as phenols, and their function as antioxidants has been well-documented. Cranberries are SUPER BENEFICIAL for Blood Type B individuals, especially non-secretors, who have a higher than average risk for urinary tract infections.

An item's value also applies to its juice, unless otherwise noted.

BLOOD TYPE B: FRUITS AND FRUIT JUICES			
Portion: 1 cup			
	African	Caucasian	Asian
Secretor	2–4	3–5	3–5
Non-Secretor	2–3	2–3	2–3
		Times per day	

SUPER BENEFICIAL	BENEFICIAL	NEUTRAL: Allowed Frequently	NEUTRAL: Allowed Infrequently	AVOID
Cranberry	Banana	Apple	Apricot	Avocado
Elderberry (dark blue/ purple)	Grape	Blackberry	Asian pear	Bitter melon
	Papaya	Blueberry	Breadfruit	Coconut
	Pineapple	Boysen- berry	Cantaloupe	Persimmon
Plum		Canang melon	Currant	Pomegranate
Watermelon		Casaba melon	Date	Prickly pear
		Cherry (all)	Fig (dried/ fresh)	Star fruit (carambola)
		Christmas melon	Honeydew melon	
		Crenshaw melon	Plantain	
		Dewberry	Raisin	
		Gooseberry		
		Grapefruit		
		Guava		
		Kiwi		
		Kumquat		
		Lemon		
		Lime		
		Loganberry		
		Mango		
		Mulberry		
		Muskmelon		
		Nectarine		
		Orange		
		Peach		
		Pear		
		Persian melon		
		Prune		

SUPER BENEFICIAL	BENEFICIAL	NEUTRAL: Allowed Frequently	NEUTRAL: Allowed Infrequently	AVOID
		Quince		
		Raspberry		
		Sago palm		
		Spanish melon		
		Strawberry		
		Tangerine		
		Youngberry		

Special Variants: *Non-Secretor* BENEFICIAL: blackberry, blueberry, boysenberry, cherry, currant, elderberry (dark blue/purple), fig (dried/fresh), guava, raspberry; NEUTRAL (Allowed Frequently): banana; AVOID: cantaloupe, honeydew.

Spices/Condiments/Sweeteners

Many spices are known to have medicinal properties. Turmeric improves liver function. Ginger aids digestive health, as does cayenne pepper. Licorice provides antiviral support and is important in effectively processing cortisol. Many common food additives, such as guar gum and carrageenan, enhance the effects of lectins found in other foods and should be avoided. Use caution when using prepared condiments. Often they contain wheat.

SUPER BENEFICIAL	BENEFICIAL	NEUTRAL: Allowed Frequently	NEUTRAL: Allowed Infrequently	AVOID
Ginger	Horse-radish	Anise	Agar	Allspice
Licorice root*	Molasses (black-strap)	Apple pectin	Arrowroot	Almond extract
Pepper (cayenne)	Parsley	Basil	Chocolate	Aspartame
Turmeric		Bay leaf	Fructose	Barley malt
		Bergamot	Honey	Carrageenan
		Caper	Maple syrup	Cinnamon

SUPER BENEFICIAL	BENEFICIAL	NEUTRAL: Allowed Frequently	NEUTRAL: Allowed Infrequently	AVOID
		Caraway	Mayonnaise	Cornstarch
		Cardamom	Molasses	Corn syrup
		Carob	Pickles (all)	Dextrose
		Chervil	Rice syrup	Gelatin (except veg-sourced)
		Chili powder	Sugar (brown/white)	Guarana
		Chive	Tamari (wheat-free)	Gums (acacia/Arabic/guar)
		Cilantro (coriander leaf)	Vinegar (all)	Juniper
		Clove		Ketchup
		Coriander		Malto-dextrin
		Cream of tartar		MSG
		Cumin		Pepper (black/white)
		Dill		Soy sauce
		Fenugreek		Stevia
		Garlic		Sucanat
		Lecithin		Tapioca
		Mace		
		Marjoram		
		Mint (all)		
		Mustard (dry)		
		Nutmeg		
		Oregano		
		Paprika		
		Pepper (pepper-corn/red flakes)		
		Rosemary		
		Saffron		

SUPER BENEFICIAL	BENEFICIAL	NEUTRAL: Allowed Frequently	NEUTRAL: Allowed Infrequently	AVOID
		Sage		
		Savory		
		Sea salt		
		Seaweeds		
		Senna		
		Tamarind		
		Tarragon		
		Thyme		
		Vanilla		
		Winter-green		
		Yeast (baker's/ brewer's)		

Special Variants: *Non-Secretor* BENEFICIAL: oregano, yeast (brewer's); NEUTRAL (Allowed Frequently): stevia; AVOID: agar, fructose, pickle relish, sugar (brown/white).

*Not to be used if you have high blood pressure.

Herbal Teas

Several herbal teas are SUPER BENEFICIAL for Blood Type B. Ginger contains pungent phenolic substances with pronounced antioxidative and anti-inflammatory activities. Sage is rich in rosmarinic acid, which acts to reduce inflammatory responses by altering the concentrations of inflammatory messaging molecules. The leaves and stems of the sage plant contain antioxidant enzymes, including superoxide dismutase (SOD) and peroxidase. When combined, these three components of sage—flavonoids, phenolic acids, and oxygen-handling enzymes—give it a unique capacity for stabilizing oxygen-related metabolism and preventing oxygen-based damage to the cells. Licorice root tea provides antiviral support for Blood Type B. Ginseng and dandelion can help reduce stress.

SUPER BENEFICIAL	BENEFICIAL	NEUTRAL: Allowed Frequently	NEUTRAL: Allowed Infrequently	AVOID
Dandelion	Parsley	Alfalfa	Dong quai	Aloe
Ginger	Pepper-	Burdock		Coltsfoot
Ginseng	mint	Catnip		Corn silk
Licorice	Raspberry	Chamomile		Fenugreek
root*	leaf	Chickweed		Gentian
Sage	Rosehip	Echinacea		Hops
		Elder		Linden
		Goldenseal		Mullein
		Hawthorn		Red clover
		Horehound		Rhubarb
		Mulberry		Shepherd's
		Rosemary		purse
		Sarsaparilla		Skullcap
		Senna		
		Slippery elm		
		Spearmint		
		St. John's wort		
		Strawberry leaf		
		Thyme		
		Valerian		
		Vervain		
		White birch		
		White oak bark		
		Yarrow		
		Yellow dock		

Special Variants: None.

*Not to be used if you have high blood pressure.

Miscellaneous Beverages

Green tea should be part of every Blood Type B's health plan. It contains polyphenols, which enhance gastrointestinal health. Alcohol can exacerbate autoimmune inflammatory conditions. Limit alcohol to an occasional glass of red wine. If you are a heavy coffee drinker, try to reduce your intake or slowly eliminate it altogether.

SUPER BENEFICIAL	BENEFICIAL	NEUTRAL: Allowed Frequently	NEUTRAL: Allowed Infrequently	AVOID
Tea (green)		Wine (red/white)	Beer	Liquor
			Coffee (reg/decaf)	Seltzer
				Soda (club)
			Tea, black (reg/decaf)	Soda (cola/diet/misc.)

Special Variants: *Non-Secretor* BENEFICIAL: wine (red/white); NEUTRAL (Allowed Frequently): liquor, seltzer, soda (club); AVOID: coffee (reg/decaf), tea, black (reg/decaf).

Supplements

THE BLOOD TYPE B DIET offers abundant quantities of important nutrients, such as protein and iron. It is important to get as many nutrients as possible from fresh foods and use supplements only to fill in the minor deficiencies in your diet. The following supplement protocols are designed for Blood Type B individuals who are suffering from conditions that cause fatigue.

Note: If you are being treated for a medical condition, consult your doctor before taking any supplements.

Blood Type B: Basic Fatigue Protocol

Use this protocol for 4–8 weeks, then discontinue for 2 weeks and restart.

SUPPLEMENT	ACTION	DOSAGE
Magnesium citrate	Essential for nerve and digestive health.	250 mg: 2 capsules, twice daily
High-potency vitamin-mineral complex (preferably blood type–specific)	Nutritional support.	As directed
High-quality "green drink"	Typically includes a wide variety of sprouted seeds and grasses with high nutritional integrity and enzymatic activity. May also contain antioxidant-rich foods.	As directed
Vinpocetine	Experiments with vinpocetine indicate that it can enhance circulation in the brain, improve oxygen utilization, make red blood cells more pli-able, and inhibit aggre-gation of platelets.	10 mg, twice daily

Blood Type B: Immune System Health Maintenance

Use this protocol for 4–8 weeks, then discontinue for 2 weeks and restart.

SUPPLEMENT	ACTION	DOSAGE
Gokharu/Caltrop (*Tribulus terrestris*) fruit extract; 20% furanosterols	Improves strength and protection against infection.	50 mg: 1–2 capsules daily

SUPPLEMENT	ACTION	DOSAGE
Maitake extract (*Grifola frondosa*)	Improves immune function.	500 mg: 2–3 capsules, twice daily
Carob (*Ceratonia siliqua*)	Useful for nervous exhaustion.	Solid extract: ¼– ½ tsp, twice daily
Eucommia bark (*Cortex eucommiae*)	Traditionally used in Chinese medicine for nourishing the liver and kidney and strengthening the bones and muscles.	10–15 g, decocted in water, twice daily

Blood Type B: Stress Management

Use this protocol for 4–8 weeks, then discontinue for 2 weeks and restart.

SUPPLEMENT	ACTION	DOSAGE
NADH (nicotinamide adenine dinucleotide)	NADH, through a series of reactions with acetyl and oxygen, is able to produce energy. This energy is in the form of ATP (adenosine triphosphate).	5-mg tablet a few times a week in the morning, on an empty stomach, with water. Wait 10–30 minutes before eating.
Siberian ginseng (*Eleutherococcus senticosus*)	Increases energy and stamina; adaptogen.	250 mg: 1 capsule, twice daily
Holy basil (*Ocimum sanctum*)	Recent studies have shown that it affords significant protection against stress.	Tincture or herbal glycerite: 15 drops in warm water, twice daily

Blood Type B: Addressing Metabolic or Environmental Toxicities

Use this protocol for 4–8 weeks, then discontinue for 2 weeks and restart.

SUPPLEMENT	ACTION	DOSAGE
Sprouted food complex, preferably made from B BENEFICIALS	Enhances detoxification.	1–2 capsules, twice daily
Probiotic (preferably blood type–specific)	Promotes intestinal health.	1–2 capsules, twice daily
Larch arabinogalactan	Promotes digestive and intestinal health.	1 tablespoon, twice daily, in juice or water
Green tea	Supports cardiovascular and immune system health.	1–3 cups daily

Blood Type B: Cellular Blockage

Use this protocol for 4–8 weeks, then discontinue for 2 weeks and restart.

SUPPLEMENT	ACTION	DOSAGE
L-arginine	Facilitates immune function and increases nitric oxide synthesis.	250 mg: 1–2 capsules, twice daily
Licorice (*Glycyrrhiza* sp)*	Supports liver function. Licorice contains glycyrrhizin, which is absorbed as glycyrrhetinic acid. Glycyrrhizin inhibits an enzyme called 11-beta-hydroxysteroid dehydrogenase, which converts cortisol to cortisone.	1 cup of tea, twice daily, or herbal preparations under direction of a physician

SUPPLEMENT	ACTION	DOSAGE
Potassium citrate	Necessary for proper protein and carbohydrate metabolism; synergistic with licorice.	99 mg: 1 capsule, twice daily

*Licorice can cause sodium and water retention. It should be used with a potassium supplement or in conjunction with a high-potassium diet.

The Exercise Component

FOR BLOOD TYPE B, stress regulation and overall fitness are achieved with a balance of moderate aerobic activity and mentally soothing, stress-reducing exercises. Below is a list of exercises that are recommended for Blood Type B.

EXERCISE	DURATION	FREQUENCY
Tennis	45–60 minutes	2–3 x week
Martial arts	30–60 minutes	2–3 x week
Cycling	45–60 minutes	2–3 x week
Hiking	30–60 minutes	2–3 x week
Golf (no cart!)	60–90 minutes	2–3 x week
Running or brisk walking	40–50 minutes	2–3 x week
Pilates	40–50 minutes	2–3 x week
Swimming	45 minutes	2–3 x week
Hatha yoga	40–50 minutes	1–2 x week
T'ai Chi	40–50 minutes	1–2 x week

3 Steps to Effective Exercise

1. Warm up with stretching and flexibility moves before you start your aerobic exercise.
2. To achieve maximum cardiovascular benefits, work toward an elevated heart rate that is about 70 percent of your capacity. Once you reach the elevated rate, continue exercis-

ing to maintain that rate for twenty to thirty minutes. To calculate your maximum heart rate and performance level:

- Subtract your age from 220.
- Multiply the difference by .70 (or .60 if you are over age sixty). This is the high end of your performance.
- Multiply the remainder by .50. This is the low end of your performance.

3. Finish each aerobic session with at least a five-minute cooldown of stretching and relaxation moves.

Getting Started: The First Month

If you are new to the Blood Type Diet, the following guidelines will introduce you to the Blood Type B regimen over a period of one month. Follow these recommendations as closely as possible, using a notebook to record your personal experiences with the diet. In addition to factors that are measurable in laboratory tests, take the time to note changes in your energy levels, sleep patterns, digestion, and overall well-being.

Blood Type B Fatigue-Fighting Diet Checklist

Eat small-to-moderate portions of high-quality, lean, organic ☐ meat (especially goat, lamb, and mutton) several times a week for strength, energy, and digestive health.

Avoid chicken. ☐

Include regular portions of richly oiled cold-water fish. ☐

Regularly eat cultured dairy foods, such as yogurt and kefir, ☐ which are beneficial for digestive health.

Eliminate wheat and corn from your diet. ☐

Eat lots of BENEFICIAL fruits and vegetables. ☐

If you need a daily dose of caffeine, replace coffee with ☐
green tea.

Avoid foods that are Type B red flags, especially chicken, ☐
corn, buckwheat, peanuts, soy beans, lentils, potatoes, and
tomatoes.

Week 1

Blood Type Diet and Supplements

- Eliminate your most harmful AVOID foods—chicken, corn, and wheat.
- Include your most important BENEFICIAL foods on a regular schedule throughout the week. For example, have lean red meat 5 times, and omega-3-rich fish 3 to 4 times, with lots of BENEFICIAL vegetables and fruit.
- Incorporate at least 1 SUPER BENEFICIAL into your daily diet. For example, have a handful of walnuts as a snack, or eat yogurt mixed with berries for lunch.
- If you're a coffee drinker, begin to wean yourself by cutting your daily consumption in half, substituting green tea.

Exercise Regimen

- Plan to exercise at least 4 days this week, for 45 minutes each day.

  2–3 days: aerobic activity

  1–2 days: Hatha yoga or T'ai Chi
- If you have an infection or are in ill health, start slowly and gradually increase your duration and intensity of activity. The important factor is consistency. Just do it—as much as you're able.
- Use your journal to detail the time, activity, distance, and amount of weight lifted. Note the number of repetitions for each exercise.

▪ WEEK 1 SUCCESS STRATEGY ▪
Stimulate without Stimulants

If you crave any form of stimulants or carbohydrates, your serotonin
levels are probably low, and your brain is demanding stimulants
to raise your serotonin levels. Try drinking some unsweetened
cocoa powder in hot water or in a whey protein smoothie. Small
amounts of serotonin are in chocolate, which explains why we feel

so good when we eat it. Try a sip of vegetable glycerine between meals to cut down on your cravings. Avoid using the "herbal serotonin" supplements, such as 5HTP.

Week 2

Blood Type Diet and Supplements

- Begin to eliminate the next level of AVOID foods—seeds, beans, and legumes that have negative lectin activity.
- Eat at least 2 to 3 BENEFICIAL animal proteins every day from the meat, seafood, and dairy lists.
- Initially, it is best to avoid foods on the list NEUTRAL: Allowed Infrequently.
- Continue to incorporate SUPER BENEFICIAL foods into your daily diet.
- If you're a coffee drinker, continue to cut your coffee intake, replacing it with green tea.

Exercise Regimen

- Continue to exercise at least 4 days this week, for 45 minutes each day.
  2–3 days: aerobic activity
  1–2 days: Hatha yoga or T'ai Chi
- If your work is sedentary, get in the habit of taking a couple of "movement" breaks during the day. Walk around the block or up and down stairs.

■ WEEK 2 SUCCESS STRATEGY ■
Medicine in Mushrooms

Exotic mushrooms are used in traditional Chinese medicine for many health benefits. Shiitake, maitake, cordyceps, and reishi mushrooms contain compounds classified as host defense potentiators. These compounds improve immune defenses, aid neuron transmission, and regulate metabolism. They are particularly valuable for Blood Type B in building long-term antiviral resistance.

Week 3

Blood Type Diet and Supplements

- When you plan your meals for week 3, choose BENEFICIAL foods to replace NEUTRAL foods whenever possible. For example, choose lamb over beef, or blueberries over an apple.
- Eliminate all remaining AVOID foods.
- Liberally incorporate SUPER BENEFICIAL foods into your daily diet.

Exercise Regimen

- Continue to exercise at least 4 days this week, for 45 minutes each day.

  2–3 days: aerobic activity

  1–2 days: Hatha yoga or T'ai Chi

■ **WEEK 3 SUCCESS STRATEGY** ■
Visualize Your Way to a Better Immune System

Take advantage of Blood Type B's natural ability to relieve stress through meditation or guided imagery. I've never medicated Type B individuals who have high blood pressure without first teaching them some simple visualization techniques and sending them home to try them out for a few weeks. Those that did almost never required medication.

Here is a very simple visualization exercise to help control high blood pressure. Do this visualization two to four times daily for five to eight minutes.

Find a quiet place and make yourself comfortable and re-laxed. Close your eyes and let your arms and hands lie limply on your sides or in your lap. Take a few deep breaths, inhaling through your nose and exhaling through your mouth, while imagining the red blood cells of your circulatory system coursing through your arteries and veins. See them slipping and sliding along the walls, which periodically open up like Venetian blinds to allow cells to move from the inside of the arteries out and from the outside in. Imagine the walls of your arteries relaxing and bending. Now expand the image and visualize your entire body. See the blood circulating from your heart to the arteries, to the capillaries, to the veins, then back to the lungs and heart.

Week 4

Blood Type Diet and Supplements

- Continue at the week 3 level, focusing on BENEFICIAL and SUPER BENEFICIAL foods.
- Evaluate the first 4 weeks and make adjustments.

Exercise Regimen

- Continue at the week 3 level.
- Review your progress, noting in your journal improvements in strength and flexibility. Determine which exercise regimen has worked for you, including time of day, setting, and activity level.

■ **WEEK 4 SUCCESS STRATEGY** ■
Chi Breathing

Chi breathing is based upon the Taoist concept of Chi Gong, which represents energy as flowing according to certain routes in your body. Positive release is accessible through refining the breath. The calming, stress-relieving effects of this exercise are remarkable. It can be performed by anyone, regardless of age, fitness, or medical condition.

1. Stand comfortably, feet shoulder-width apart, knees slightly bent, arms at your side. Relax your neck and shoulder muscles and focus in on your solar plexus (center of the body). It is okay to sway a bit—that's normal.
2. Start to rock back and forth gently. Inhale deeply as you rock forward onto the balls of your feet; exhale as you rock backward onto your heels.
3. As you inhale, lift your relaxed arms up and forward, keeping them relaxed and slightly bent. As you exhale, let your arms float down. Imagine that your hands are pulsing around an imaginary ball of energy.
4. Repeat, gradually refining the rhythm and developing the ability to "drop" your breath from the lungs to the solar plexus.

5. Repeat four to five times, then relax, letting your hands drop to your sides and closing your eyes. Concentrate on feeling relaxed and centered.

A Final Word

IN SUMMARY, the secret to fighting fatigue with the Blood Type B Diet involves:

1. Maximizing overall health by adhering to a balanced diet that includes BENEFICIAL meat, seafood, and dairy.
2. Minimizing the consumption of toxic lectins, most abundant in chicken and in grains such as wheat, buckwheat, and corn.
3. Enhancing detoxification and elimination to increase liver efficiency and inhibit provocation of the immune system by infectious agents.
4. Using supplements intelligently to improve digestive health, reduce stress, provide antioxidant support, and balance immune function.

SIX

Blood Type

AB

BLOOD TYPE AB DIET OUTCOME: A MORNING PERSON

"I have been following the Blood Type AB Diet for only a short time, but the change in my energy is remarkable. I was having sleeping problems, along with lack of concentration and much fatigue. With my higher energy, making my own meals is easier. I have been waking and walking in the morning every day, and you have no idea how out of character this is. I have never before considered myself a 'morning person.'"

BLOOD TYPE AB DIET OUTCOME: IT FEELS RIGHT

"I have been suffering from many health problems for the past five years, and they have become increasingly worse over the past two. The most prevalent are a digestive disorder that was moderate to severe, weight that I could not lose even with the most extreme diets and exercise, and severe exhaustion. I spent many hours with my doctors, and they just assumed that I was not trying as hard as I said I was. After six weeks on the Blood Type Diet, I feel like an entirely new person. I have had no digestive problems, I have an energy level I did not know was possible for me, and I have begun losing weight. The part I like about my weight loss is that it feels like a healthy loss. I am not tired or hungry. My improvement is so great that my husband (who thinks tofu is a four-letter word) has started to encourage me to make meals that are conducive to my diet."

Self-reported outcomes from the Blood Type Diet Web site (www.dadamo.com)

Blood Type AB: The Foods

THE BLOOD TYPE AB Fatigue Diet is specifically adapted to provide the maximum nutritional support to fight fatigue. A new category, **Super Beneficial**, highlights powerful disease-fighting foods for Blood Type AB. The **Neutral** category has also been adjusted to de-emphasize foods that are less advantageous for you. Foods designated **Neutral: Allowed Infrequently** should be minimized or avoided entirely.

Your secretor status can influence your ability to fully digest and metabolize certain foods, so various adjustments in the values are made for non-secretors. If you do not know your secretor type, the odds are that you can safely use the "secretor" values, since the majority of the population (approximately 80 percent) are secretors. However, I urge you to get tested, since the variations are important for non-secretors who want to maximize the effectiveness of the Blood Type Diet. (To find out how to get tested, visit our Web site (www. dadamo.com).

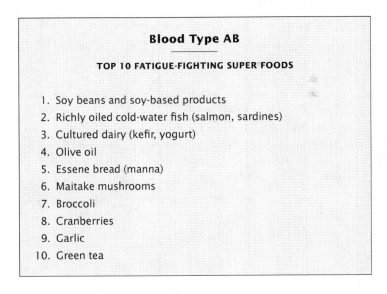

Blood Type AB

TOP 10 FATIGUE-FIGHTING SUPER FOODS

1. Soy beans and soy-based products
2. Richly oiled cold-water fish (salmon, sardines)
3. Cultured dairy (kefir, yogurt)
4. Olive oil
5. Essene bread (manna)
6. Maitake mushrooms
7. Broccoli
8. Cranberries
9. Garlic
10. Green tea

The food charts are divided into three sections. The top of the chart suggests the average portion size and quantity per week or day, according to secretor status. These recommendations do *not* apply to the category **Neutral: Allowed Infrequently;** those foods should be eaten rarely, if at all. The charts also indicate differences in frequency for some foods based on ethnic heritage. It has been my experience that this factor has an impact upon the individual's ability to fully digest certain foods. For the purposes of blood type food choices, persons of Hispanic heritage should follow the guidelines for Caucasians, and American Native peoples should follow the guidelines for Asians.

The middle section of the chart gives the food values. The bottom section lists variants based on secretor status.

For your convenience, we have included a number of product names (Ezekiel 4:9 bread, Worcestershire sauce, etc.). However, keep in mind that commercial formulations vary among brands and regions. Even though a product may be listed as acceptable for you, always check its ingredients. Some products contain **Avoid** ingredients for your blood type. Of course, you may choose to make your own version of commercial products, such as bread and mayonnaise, using ingredients that suit your blood type. There are hundreds of delicious recipes for every blood type available on our Web site (www.dadamo.com) and in the book *Cook Right 4 Your Type: The Practical Kitchen Companion to Eat Right 4 Your Type.*

Meat/Poultry

Blood Type AB is somewhat better adapted to animal-based proteins than Blood Type A, mainly because of the B gene's effects on the production of enzymes involved in fat transport and digestion. However, Type AB should limit meat and avoid chicken, which contains a B-immunoreactive lectin. Choose only the best quality (preferably free-range) chemical-, antibiotic-, and pesticide-free low-fat meats and poultry.

BLOOD TYPE AB: MEAT/POULTRY

Portion: 4–6 oz (men); 2–5 oz (women and children)

	African	Caucasian	Asian
Secretor	2–5	1–5	1–5
Non-Secretor	3–5	2–5	2–5
		Times per week	

SUPER BENEFICIAL	BENEFICIAL	NEUTRAL: Allowed Frequently	NEUTRAL: Allowed Infrequently	AVOID
	Lamb	Goat	Liver (calf)	All commercially processed meats
	Mutton	Ostrich		Bacon/ham/ pork
	Rabbit	Pheasant		Beef
	Turkey			Buffalo
				Chicken
				Cornish hen
				Duck
				Goose
				Grouse
				Guinea hen
				Heart (beef)
				Horse
				Partridge
				Quail
				Squab
				Squirrel
				Sweetbreads
				Turtle
				Veal
				Venison

Special Variants: *Non-Secretor* NEUTRAL (Allowed Frequently): quail, venison.

Fish/Seafood

Fish and seafood provide an excellent means of optimizing NK cell activity. Richly oiled cold-water fish, such as mackerel, salmon, and sardines, are good sources of omega-3 fatty acids. They are also good food sources of phosphorus and adenosine, used to make cellular energy. In general, many of the seafoods Blood Type AB must avoid have lectins with either A or B specificity, or polyamines commonly found in the foods. Avoid consuming flash-frozen fish, which has high polyamine content.

BLOOD TYPE AB: FISH/SEAFOOD			
Portion: 4–6 oz (men); 2–5 oz (women and children)			
	African	Caucasian	Asian
Secretor	4–6	3–5	3–5
Non-Secretor	4–7	4–6	4–6
	Times per week		

SUPER BENEFICIAL	BENEFICIAL	NEUTRAL: Allowed Frequently	NEUTRAL: Allowed Infrequently	AVOID
Mackerel	Cod	Abalone	Caviar	Anchovy
Salmon	Grouper	Bluefish	(sturgeon)	Barracuda
Sardine	Mahi-mahi	Bullhead	Mussel	Bass (all)
	Monkfish	Butterfish	Scallop	Beluga
	Pickerel	Carp	Squid	Clam
	Pike	Catfish	(calamari)	Conch
	Porgy	Chub	Whitefish	Crab
	Red	Croaker		Eel
	snapper	Cusk		Flounder
	Sailfish	Drum		Frog
	Shad	Halfmoon		Gray sole
	Snail (*Helix*	fish		Haddock
	pomatia/			Hake
	escargot)			

SUPER BENEFICIAL	BENEFICIAL	NEUTRAL: Allowed Frequently	NEUTRAL: Allowed Infrequently	AVOID
	Sturgeon	Harvest fish		Halibut
	Tuna	Herring (fresh)		Herring (pickled/ smoked)
		Mullet		Lobster
		Muskellunge		Octopus
		Opaleye		Oysters
		Orange roughy		Salmon (smoked)
		Parrot fish		Salmon roe
		Perch (all)		Shrimp
		Pollock		Sole
		Pompano		Trout (all)
		Rosefish		Whiting
		Scrod		Yellowtail
		Scup		
		Shark		
		Smelt		
		Sucker		
		Sunfish		
		Swordfish		
		Tilapia		
		Tilefish		
		Tuna		
		Weakfish		

Special Variants: *Non-Secretor* BENEFICIAL: herring (fresh); NEUTRAL (Allowed Frequently): trout (all).

Dairy/Eggs

Dairy products can be used with discretion by many Blood Type AB individuals, especially secretors. Cultured dairy foods, such as yogurt and kefir, are particularly BENEFICIAL. Ghee (clarified butter) is an antioxidant, rich in omega-3 oils and short-chain fatty acids. Eggs, which, like fish, are a good source of docosahexaenoic acid, can complement the protein profile for your blood type. Do your best to find eggs and dairy products that are both hormone-free and organic.

BLOOD TYPE AB: EGGS			
Portion: 1 egg			
	African	Caucasian	Asian
Secretor	2–5	3–4	3–4
Non-Secretor	3–6	3–6	3–6
		Times per week	

BLOOD TYPE AB: MILK AND YOGURT			
Portion: 4–6 oz (men); 2–5 oz (women and children)			
	African	Caucasian	Asian
Secretor	2–6	3–6	1–6
Non-Secretor	0–3	0–4	0–3
		Times per week	

BLOOD TYPE AB: CHEESE			
Portion: 3 oz (men); 2 oz (women and children)			
	African	Caucasian	Asian
Secretor	2–3	3–4	3–4
Non-Secretor	0	0–1	0
		Times per week	

SUPER BENEFICIAL	BENEFICIAL	NEUTRAL: Allowed Frequently	NEUTRAL: Allowed Infrequently	AVOID
Ghee (clarified butter)	Cottage cheese	Casein	Cheddar	American cheese
Kefir	Egg (chicken)	Cream cheese	Colby	Blue cheese
Yogurt	Farmer cheese	Edam	Emmenthal	Brie
	Feta	Egg (goose/quail)	Milk (cow)	Butter
	Goat cheese	Gouda	Monterey Jack	Buttermilk
	Milk (goat)	Gruyère	Sherbet	Camembert
	Mozzarella	Jarlsberg	Swiss cheese	Egg (duck)
	Ricotta	Muenster		Half-and-half
	Sour cream	Neufchâtel		Ice cream
		Paneer		Parmesan
		Quark		Provolone
		String cheese		
		Whey		

Special Variants: *Non-Secretor* BENEFICIAL: ghee (clarified butter); NEUTRAL (Allowed Frequently): goat cheese, yogurt; AVOID: Emmenthal, Swiss cheese.

Oils

Olive oil, a monounsaturated fat, is SUPER BENEFICIAL for Blood Type AB. Constituents in olive oil, such as flavonoids, squalenes, and polyphenols, act as powerful antioxidants. It should be used as a primary cooking oil.

Corn, sesame, and safflower oils can contain immunoreactive proteins that impair Blood Type AB digestion. These oils can interfere with proper immune function.

BLOOD TYPE AB: OILS			
Portion: 1 tblsp			
	African	**Caucasian**	**Asian**
Secretor	4–7	5–8	5–7
Non-Secretor	3–6	3–6	3–4
		Times per week	

SUPER BENEFICIAL	BENEFICIAL	NEUTRAL: Allowed Frequently	NEUTRAL: Allowed Infrequently	AVOID
Olive	Flax (linseed) Walnut	Almond Black currant seed Borage seed Canola Castor Cod liver Evening primrose Peanut Soy	Wheat germ	Coconut Corn Cottonseed Safflower Sesame Sunflower
Special Variants: None.				

Nuts and Seeds

Nuts and seeds can be an important secondary source of protein for Blood Type AB. Laboratory research has identified at least five natural phytochemicals in nuts that regulate the immune system and act as antioxidants. SUPER BENEFICIAL for Blood Type AB are flax (linseeds) and walnuts, which are high in omega-3 fatty acids.

BLOOD TYPE AB: NUTS AND SEEDS

Portion: Whole (handful); Nut Butters (2 tblsp)

	African	Caucasian	Asian
Secretor	5–10	5–10	5–9
Non-Secretor	4–8	4–9	5–9
		Times per week	

SUPER BENEFICIAL	BENEFICIAL	NEUTRAL: Allowed Frequently	NEUTRAL: Allowed Infrequently	AVOID
Flax	Chestnut	Almond	Brazil nut	Filbert (hazelnut)
Walnut (black/ English)	Peanut	Almond butter	Cashew	Poppy seed
	Peanut butter	Almond cheese	Cashew butter	Pumpkin seed
		Almond milk	Macadamia	Sesame butter (tahini)
		Beechnut	Pecan	Sesame seed
		Butternut	Pecan butter	Sunflower butter
		Hickory	Pistachio	Sunflower seed
		Litchi	Safflower seed	
		Pignolia (pine nut)		

Special Variants: *Non-Secretor* NEUTRAL (Allowed Frequently): peanut, peanut butter; AVOID: Brazil nut, cashew, cashew butter, pistachio.

Beans and Legumes

Blood Type AB does well on proteins found in many beans and legumes, although this food category contains more than a few beans with problematic A- or B-specific lectins. In general, soy beans and their related products are SUPER BENEFICIAL for the Blood Type AB immune system.

BLOOD TYPE AB: BEANS AND LEGUMES

Portion: 1 cup (cooked)

	African	Caucasian	Asian
Secretor	3–6	3–6	4–6
Non-Secretor	2–5	2–5	3–6
		Times per week	

SUPER BENEFICIAL	BENEFICIAL	NEUTRAL: Allowed Frequently	NEUTRAL: Allowed Infrequently	AVOID
Soy bean	Lentil	Bean	Jicama	Adzuki bean
Soy cheese	(green)	(green/	bean	Black bean
Soy milk	Navy bean	snap/		Black-eyed
Soy, miso	Pinto bean	string)		pea
Soy,		Cannellini		Fava (broad)
tempeh		bean		bean
Soy, tofu		Copper		Garbanzo
		bean		(chickpea)
		Lentil		Kidney bean
		(domestic/		Lima bean
		red)		Mung bean/
		Northern		sprout
		bean		
		Pea (green/		
		pod/		
		snow)		
		Tamarind		
		bean		
		White bean		

Special Variants: *Non-Secretor* NEUTRAL (Allowed Frequently): fava (broad) bean, navy bean, soy bean, soy (miso), soy (tempeh), soy (tofu); AVOID: jicama bean, soy cheese, soy milk.

Grains and Starches

Blood Type AB benefits from a moderate consumption of the proper grains for its blood type. Essene bread (manna) is SUPER BENEFICIAL. It is a 100-percent sprouted bread, from which the lectin-containing seed coat has been removed. Blood Type AB individuals—especially non-secretors—should use Essene instead of other wheat breads. Blood Type AB is also sensitive to the lectin in corn and should avoid all corn flour products.

BLOOD TYPE AB: GRAINS AND STARCHES			
Portion: ½ cup dry (grains or pastas); 1 muffin; 2 slices of bread			
	African	**Caucasian**	**Asian**
Secretor	6–8	6–9	6–10
Non-Secretor	4–6	5–7	6–8
			Times per week

SUPER BENEFICIAL	BENEFICIAL	NEUTRAL: Allowed Frequently	NEUTRAL: Allowed Infrequently	AVOID
Essene bread (manna)	Amaranth Ezekiel 4:9 bread Millet Oat bran Oat flour Oatmeal Rice (whole) Rice (wild) Rice bran	Barley Couscous Quinoa Spelt flour/ products	Wheat (semolina) Wheat (whole) Wheat bran Wheat germ	Buckwheat Cornmeal Grits Kamut Popcorn Soba noodles (100% buckwheat) Sorghum Tapioca Teff

SUPER BENEFICIAL	BENEFICIAL	NEUTRAL: Allowed Frequently	NEUTRAL: Allowed Infrequently	AVOID
	Rice cake Rye (whole) Rye flour/ products Soy flour/ products Spelt (whole)			Wheat (refined/ unbleached) Wheat (white flour)

Special Variants: *Non-Secretor* NEUTRAL (Allowed Frequently): Ezekiel 4:9 bread, spelt (whole); AVOID: soy flour/products, wheat (semolina), wheat (whole), wheat germ.

Vegetables

Vegetables can be your first line of defense against chronic disease. They provide a rich source of antioxidants and fiber and are essential to intestinal health. Blood Type AB SUPER BENEFICIALS include onions, which are high in quercetin, a flavonoid with potent anti-inflammatory properties, and other antioxidants that decrease oxidative stress and increase glutathione, which protects cells. Broccoli is a potent antioxidant. Mushrooms (maitake and the common domestic variety, called silver dollar) are powerful infection fighters. Cabbage—especially the juice—and cauliflower are detoxifying for Blood Type AB.

An item's value also applies to its juice, unless otherwise noted.

BLOOD TYPE AB: VEGETABLES

Portion: 1 cup, prepared (cooked or raw)

	African	Caucasian	Asian
Secretor Super/ Beneficials	Unlimited	Unlimited	Unlimited
Secretor Neutrals	2–5	2–5	2–5
Non-Secretor Super/ Beneficials	Unlimited	Unlimited	Unlimited
Non-Secretor Neutrals	2–3	2–3	2–3
	Times per day		

SUPER BENEFICIAL	BENEFICIAL	NEUTRAL: Allowed Frequently	NEUTRAL: Allowed Infrequently	AVOID
Broccoli	Alfalfa	Arugula	Carrot	Aloe
Cabbage (juice)*	sprouts	Asparagus	Daikon	Artichoke
Cauliflower	Beet	Asparagus	radish	Corn
Mushroom	Beet	pea	Olives	Mushroom
(maitake/	greens	Bamboo	(Greek/	(abalone/
silver	Carrot	shoot	green/	shiitake)
dollar)	(juice)	Bok choy	Spanish)	Olive
Onion (all)	Celery	Brussels	Poi	(black)
	Cucumber	sprouts	Potato	Peppers (all)
	Collards	Cabbage	Pumpkin	Pickles (all)
	Dandelion	Celeriac	Taro	Radish/
	Eggplant	Chicory		sprouts
	Kale	Cucumber		Rhubarb
	Mustard	(juice)		
	greens	Endive		
	Parsnip	Escarole		
	Potato	Fennel		
	(sweet)	Fiddlehead		
	Yam	fern		

SUPER BENEFICIAL	BENEFICIAL	NEUTRAL: Allowed Frequently	NEUTRAL: Allowed Infrequently	AVOID
		Horseradish		
		Kohlrabi		
		Leek		
		Lettuce (all)		
		Mushroom (enoki/ oyster/ portobello/ straw/ tree ear)		
		Okra		
		Oyster plant		
		Radicchio		
		Rappini (broccoli rabe)		
		Rutabaga		
		Scallion		
		Seaweeds		
		Shallot		
		Spinach		
		Squash (all)		
		Swiss chard		
		Tomato		
		Turnip		
		Water chestnut		

SUPER BENEFICIAL	BENEFICIAL	NEUTRAL: Allowed Frequently	NEUTRAL: Allowed Infrequently	AVOID
		Watercress Yucca Zucchini		

Special Variants: *Non-Secretor* BENEFICIAL: tomato; NEUTRAL (Allowed Frequently): beet; AVOID: poi, taro.

*To obtain the benefits of cabbage juice, it must be consumed within one minute of juicing.

Fruits and Fruit Juices

SUPER BENEFICIAL fruits for Blood Type AB include cherries, which contain pigments that inhibit intestinal toxins, and cranberries, which can help fight urinary tract infections. Many fruits, such as pineapple, are rich in enzymes that can help reduce inflammation and encourage proper water balance. Grapes and grape juice are powerful antioxidants.

An item's value also applies to its juice, unless otherwise noted.

BLOOD TYPE AB: FRUITS AND FRUIT JUICES			
Portion: 1 cup			
	African	Caucasian	Asian
Secretor	3–4	3–6	3–5
Non-Secretor	1–3	2–3	3–4
	Times per day		

SUPER BENEFICIAL	BENEFICIAL	NEUTRAL: Allowed Frequently	NEUTRAL: Allowed Infrequently	AVOID
Cherry	Fig (fresh/	Apple	Apricot	Avocado
Cranberry	dried)	Blackberry	Asian pear	Banana
Grape (all)	Gooseberry	Blueberry	Breadfruit	Bitter melon
	Grapefruit	Boysen-	Canang	Coconut
	Kiwi	berry	melon	Dewberry
	Lemon	Elderberry	Cantaloupe	Guava
	Loganberry	(dark blue/	Casaba	Mango
	Pineapple	purple)	melon	Orange
	Plum	Grapefruit	Christmas	Persimmon
	Watermelon	(juice)	melon	Pomegranate
		Kumquat	Crenshaw	Prickly pear
		Lime	melon	Quince
		Mulberry	Currant	Sago palm
		Muskmelon	Date	Star fruit
		Nectarine	Honeydew	(carambola)
		Papaya	Prune	
		Peach	Raisin	
		Pear	Tangerine	
		Persian		
		melon		
		Pineapple		
		(juice)		
		Plantain		
		Raspberry		
		Spanish		
		melon		
		Strawberry		
		Youngberry		

Special Variants: *Non-Secretor* BENEFICIAL: blackberry, blueberry, elderberry (dark blue/purple), lime; NEUTRAL (Allowed Frequently): banana; AVOID: cantaloupe, honeydew, prune, tangerine.

Spices/Condiments/Sweeteners

Many spices have medicinal properties. Turmeric improves liver function. Ginger is anti-inflammatory and aids digestive health. Garlic improves immune health and is anti-inflammatory.

Many common food additives, such as guar gum and carrageenan, enhance the effects of lectins found in other foods and should be avoided.

SUPER BENEFICIAL	BENEFICIAL	NEUTRAL: Allowed Frequently	NEUTRAL: Allowed Infrequently	AVOID
Garlic	Horse-	Basil	Agar	Allspice
Ginger	radish	Bay leaf	Apple	Almond
Turmeric	Molasses	Bergamot	pectin	extract
	(black-	Caraway	Arrowroot	Anise
	strap)	Cardamom	Chocolate	Aspartame
	Oregano	Carob	Honey	Barley malt
	Parsley	Chervil	Maple	Carrageenan
		Chili	syrup	Cornstarch
		powder	Mayon-	Corn
		Chive	naise	syrup
		Cilantro	Molasses	Dextrose
		(coriander	Rice syrup	Fructose
		leaf)	Senna	Gelatin
		Cinnamon	Soy sauce	(except
		Clove	Sugar	veg-
		Coriander	(brown/	sourced)
		Cream of	white)	Guarana
		tartar		Gums
		Cumin		(acacia/
		Dill		Arabic
		Juniper		guar)
		Licorice		Ketchup
		root*		Maltodex-
		Mace		trin

SUPER BENEFICIAL	BENEFICIAL	NEUTRAL: Allowed Frequently	NEUTRAL: Allowed Infrequently	AVOID
		Marjoram		MSG
		Mint (all)		Pepper (black/ white)
		Mustard (dry)		Pepper (cayenne)
		Nutmeg		Pepper (pepper- corn/red flakes)
		Paprika		
		Rosemary		
		Saffron		
		Sage		Pickle (all)
		Savory		Sucanat
		Sea salt		Tapioca
		Seaweeds		Vinegar (all)
		Stevia		Worcester- shire sauce
		Tamari (wheat- free)		
		Tamarind		
		Tarragon		
		Thyme		
		Vanilla		
		Winter- green		
		Yeast (baker's/ brewer's)		

Special Variants: *Non-Secretor* BENEFICIAL: bay leaf, yeast (brewer's); AVOID: agar, honey, juniper, maple syrup, rice syrup, sugar (brown/white).

*Do not use if you have high blood pressure.

Herbal Teas

Several herbal teas can be SUPER BENEFICIAL for Blood Type AB. Ginger contains pungent phenolic substances with pronounced antioxidative and anti-inflammatory activities. Echinacea is mildly stimulative to the immune system. Licorice root provides antiviral support and enhances cortisol modulation.

SUPER BENEFICIAL	BENEFICIAL	NEUTRAL: Allowed Frequently	NEUTRAL: Allowed Infrequently	AVOID
Echinacea	Alfalfa	Catnip	Senna	Aloe
Ginger	Burdock	Chickweed		Coltsfoot
Licorice root*	Chamomile	Dong quai		Corn silk
	Dandelion	Elder		Fenugreek
	Ginseng	Goldenseal		Gentian
	Hawthorn	Horehound		Hops
	Parsley	Mulberry		Linden
	Rosehip	Peppermint		Mullein
	Strawberry leaf	Raspberry leaf		Red clover
		Sage		Rhubarb
		Sarsaparilla		Shepherd's purse
		Slippery elm		Skullcap
		Spearmint		
		St. John's wort		
		Thyme		
		Valerian		
		Vervain		
		White birch		

SUPER BENEFICIAL	BENEFICIAL	NEUTRAL: Allowed Frequently	NEUTRAL: Allowed Infrequently	AVOID
		White oak bark Yarrow Yellow dock		

Special Variants: None.

*Do not use if you have high blood pressure.

Miscellaneous Beverages

Green tea is a SUPER BENEFICIAL beverage for Blood Type A because of its antioxidant and cardiovascular properties. Red wine contains gallic acid, trans-resveratrol, quercetin, and rutin—four phenolic compounds with potent antioxidant effects. Coffee should be avoided by Type AB as it exacerbates allergies.

SUPER BENEFICIAL	BENEFICIAL	NEUTRAL: Allowed Frequently	NEUTRAL: Allowed Infrequently	AVOID
Tea (green)	Wine (red)	Seltzer Soda (club) Wine (white)	Beer	Coffee (reg/ decaf) Liquor Soda (cola/diet/ misc.) Tea, black (reg/ decaf)

Special Variants: *Non-Secretor* AVOID: beer.

Supplements

THE BLOOD TYPE AB DIET offers abundant quantities of important nutrients, such as protein and iron. It is important to get as many nutrients as possible from fresh foods and use supplements only to fill in the minor deficiencies in your diet. The following supplement protocols are designed for Blood Type AB individuals who are suffering from conditions that cause fatigue.

Note: If you are being treated for a medical condition, consult your doctor before taking any supplements.

Blood Type AB: Basic Fatigue Protocol

Use this protocol for 4–8 weeks, then discontinue for 2 weeks and restart.

SUPPLEMENT	ACTION	DOSAGE
Methylcobalamine (active B_{12})	Plays important role in homocysteine regulation, red blood cell production, and nerve integrity.	500 mcg daily
High-potency vitamin-mineral complex (preferably blood type–specific)	Nutritional support.	As directed
High-quality "green drink"	Typically includes a wide variety of sprouted seeds and grasses with high nutritional integrity and enzymatic activity. May also contain antioxidant rich foods.	As directed

SUPPLEMENT	ACTION	DOSAGE
Plant sterols and sterolins	A daily supplement of plant sterols and sterolins has been proven to have positive immune-balancing effects. A balanced immune system allows you to enjoy vibrant health.	"Moducare"—1–2 capsules daily

Blood Type AB: Immune System Health Maintenance

Use this protocol for 4–8 weeks, then discontinue for 2 weeks and restart.

SUPPLEMENT	ACTION	DOSAGE
Milk thistle (*Silymarin*)	*Silymarin* not only prevents the depletion of glutathione induced by alcohol and other toxic chemicals, but has been shown to increase the level of glutathione.	1–2 capsules, standardized extract, twice daily. Try to take milk thistle with a meal containing eggs. Studies have shown that when milk thistle is combined with phosphatidyl choline (found in eggs), its absorption is significantly higher.
Vitamin C (from acerola cherry or rosehips)	Acts as an antioxidant.	250 mg: 1 capsule, twice daily
Selenium	Selenium is a mineral cofactor in the manufacture of glutathione peroxidase.	50–100 mcg daily

SUPPLEMENT	ACTION	DOSAGE
Carob (*Ceratonia siliqua*)	Useful for nervous exhaustion.	Solid extract: ¼–½ tsp, twice daily

Blood Type AB: Stress Management

Use this protocol for 4–8 weeks, then discontinue for 2 weeks and restart.

SUPPLEMENT	ACTION	DOSAGE
NADH (nicotinamide adenine dinucleotide)	NADH, through a series of reactions with acetyl and oxygen, is able to produce energy. This energy is in the form of ATP (adenosine triphosphate).	5-mg tablet a few times a week in the morning, on an empty stomach, with water. Wait 10–30 minutes before eating.
Spreading hogwood (*Boerhaavia diffusa*)	*Boerhaavia diffusa* has a dramatic effect in buffering against elevation of plasma cortisol levels under stressful conditions. It also acts to reverse the depletion of adrenal cortisol associated with adrenal exhaustion.	50–100 mg daily
Holy basil (*Ocimum sanctum*)	Recent studies have shown that it affords significant protection against stress.	Tincture or herbal glycerite: 15 drops in warm water, twice daily

Blood Type AB: Addressing Metabolic or Environmental Toxicities

Use this protocol for 4–8 weeks, then discontinue for 2 weeks and restart.

SUPPLEMENT	ACTION	DOSAGE
Sprouted food complex, preferably made from AB BENEFICIALS	Enhances detoxification.	1–2 capsules, twice daily
Probiotic (preferably blood type–specific)	Promotes intestinal health.	1–2 capsules, twice daily
Larch arabinogalactan	Promotes digestive and intestinal health.	1 tablespoon, twice daily, in juice or water
Triphala—a combination of Amla (*Phyllanthus emblica*), Beleric mycrobalan (*Terminalia belerica*), and Chebulic myrobalan (*Terminalia chebula*)	Aids digestion and intestinal cleansing.	500 mg: 1 capsule, twice daily

Blood Type AB: Cellular Blockage

Use this protocol for 4–8 weeks, then discontinue for 2 weeks and restart.

SUPPLEMENT	ACTION	DOSAGE
L-arginine	Facilitates immune function and increases nitric oxide synthesis.	250 mg: 1–2 capsules, twice daily

SUPPLEMENT	ACTION	DOSAGE
Licorice (*Glycyrrhiza* sp)*	Supports liver function. Licorice contains glycyrrhizin, which is absorbed as glycyrrhetinic acid. Glycyrrhizin inhibits an enzyme called 11-beta-hydroxysteroid dehydrogenase, which converts cortisol to cortisone.	1 cup of tea, twice daily, or herbal preparations under direction of a physician
L-acetyl-cysteine (NAC)	Aids metabolic activity; substrate for glutathione production.	500 mg: 1 capsule, twice daily
Potassium citrate	Necessary for proper protein and carbohydrate metabolism; has synergies with licorice.	99 mg: 1 capsule, twice daily

*Licorice can cause sodium and water retention. It should be used with a potassium supplement or in conjunction with a high-potassium diet.

The Exercise Component

FOR BLOOD TYPE AB, overall fitness is achieved with a balance of moderate aerobic activity and mentally soothing, stress-reducing exercises. Below is a list of exercises that are recommended for Blood Type AB.

EXERCISE	DURATION	FREQUENCY
Martial arts	30–60 minutes	2–3 x week
Cycling	45–60 minutes	2–3 x week
Hiking	30–60 minutes	2–3 x week
Golf (no cart!)	60–90 minutes	2–3 x week

EXERCISE	DURATION	FREQUENCY
Walking	40–50 minutes	2–3 x week
Pilates	40–50 minutes	2–3 x week
Swimming	45 minutes	2–3 x week
Hatha Yoga	40–50 minutes	1–2 x week
T'ai Chi	40–50 minutes	1–2 x week

3 Steps to Effective Exercise

1. Warm up with stretching and flexibility moves before you start your aerobic exercise.
2. To achieve maximum cardiovascular benefits, work toward an elevated heart rate that is about 70 percent of your capacity. Once you reach the elevated rate, continue exercising to maintain that rate for twenty to thirty minutes. To calculate your maximum heart rate and performance level:
   - Subtract your age from 220.
   - Multiply the difference by .70 (or .60 if you are over age sixty). This is the high end of your performance.
   - Multiply the remainder by .50. This is the low end of your performance.
3. Finish each aerobic session with at least a five-minute cooldown of stretching and relaxation moves.

Getting Started: The First Month

IF YOU ARE NEW to the Blood Type Diet, the following guidelines will introduce you to the Blood Type AB regimen over a period of one month. Follow these recommendations as closely as possible, using a notebook to record your personal experiences with the diet. In addition to factors that are measurable in laboratory tests, take the time to note changes in your energy levels, pain levels, sleep patterns, digestion, and overall well-being.

Blood Type AB Fatigue-Fighting Diet Checklist

Derive your protein primarily from sources other than ☐ red meat.

Eliminate chicken from your diet. ☐

Eat soy foods and seafood as your primary protein. ☐

Include modest amounts of cultured dairy foods in your diet, ☐ but limit fresh milk products.

Don't overdo the grains, especially wheat-derived foods. ☐ Avoid corn flour altogether.

Eat lots of BENEFICIAL fruits and vegetables, especially those ☐ high in antioxidants and fiber.

Avoid coffee, but drink two to three cups of green tea ☐ every day.

Week 1

Blood Type Diet and Supplements

- Eliminate your most harmful AVOID foods—chicken, corn, buckwheat, most shellfish, and lectin-activated beans.
- Include your most important BENEFICIAL foods frequently throughout the week. For example, have soy-based foods 5 times, and omega-3-rich fish 3 to 4 times, with lots of BENEFICIAL vegetables and fruit.
- Incorporate at least 1 SUPER BENEFICIAL into your daily diet. For example, eat slices of fresh pineapple over yogurt, or sprinkle walnuts on a salad.
- If you're a coffee drinker, begin to wean yourself by cutting your daily consumption in half. Substitute green tea.

Exercise Regimen

- Plan to exercise at least 4 days this week, for 45 minutes each day.

  2 days: walking or light aerobic activity

  2 days: Hatha yoga or T'ai Chi
- Use your journal to detail the time, activity, distance, and amount of weight. Note the number of repetitions for each exercise.

- **WEEK 1 SUCCESS STRATEGY**
Improve Your Natural Killer Cell Activity

- Increase your intake of green vegetables.
- Increase your intake of soy bean products.
- Increase your intake of omega-3 fatty acids.
- Decrease your intake of polyunsaturated vegetable fats.
- Keep dietary fat intake between 20 and 25% of calories.
- Maintain proper body weight.
- Exercise.
- Use modest amounts of alcohol.
- Moderate your work hours.
- Don't smoke.
- Decrease stress.

Week 2

Blood Type Diet and Supplements

- Begin to eliminate the next level of AVOID foods—grains, vegetables, and fruits that react poorly with Type AB blood.
- Eat 2 to 3 BENEFICIAL proteins every day.
- Continue to incorporate SUPER BENEFICIAL foods into your daily diet.
- Choose the NEUTRAL foods listed as "Allowed Frequently" over those listed "Allowed Infrequently."
- If you're a coffee drinker, continue to cut your coffee intake, replacing it with green tea.
- Manage your mealtimes to aid proper digestion. Avoid eating on the run. Make your meals relaxing, sit-down affairs. Eat slowly and chew thoroughly to encourage digestive secretions.

Exercise Regimen

- Continue to exercise at least 4 days this week, for 45 minutes each day.

  2 days: walking or light aerobic activity

  2 days: Hatha yoga or T'ai Chi
- If your work is sedentary, get in the habit of taking a couple of "movement" breaks during the day. Walk around the block or up and down stairs.

■ **WEEK 2 SUCCESS STRATEGY** ■
Chi Breathing

Chi breathing is based upon the Taoist concept of Chi Gong, which represents energy as flowing according to certain routes in your body. Positive release is accessible through refining the breath. The calming, stress-relieving effects of this exercise are remarkable. It can be performed by anyone, regardless of age, fitness, or medical condition.

1. Stand comfortably, feet shoulder-width apart, knees slightly bent, arms at your side. Relax your neck and shoulder muscles and focus on your solar plexus (center of the body). It is okay to sway a bit—that's normal.
2. Start to rock back and forth gently. Inhale deeply as you rock forward onto the balls of your feet; exhale as you rock backward onto your heels.
3. As you inhale, lift your relaxed arms up and forward, keeping them relaxed and slightly bent. As you exhale, let your arms float down. Imagine that your hands are pulsing around an imaginary ball of energy.
4. Repeat, gradually refining the rhythm and developing the ability to "drop" your breath from the lungs to the solar plexus.
5. Repeat four to five times, then relax, letting your hands drop to your sides and closing your eyes. Concentrate on feeling relaxed and centered.

Week 3

Blood Type Diet and Supplements

- When you plan your meals for week 3, choose BENEFICIAL foods to replace NEUTRAL foods whenever possible.
- Eliminate all remaining AVOID foods.
- Liberally incorporate SUPER BENEFICIAL foods into your daily diet.
- Completely wean yourself from coffee, substituting green tea.

Exercise Regimen

- Continue to exercise at least 4 days this week, for 45 minutes each day.

  2 days: walking or light aerobic activity

  2 days: Hatha yoga or T'ai Chi

■ WEEK 3 SUCCESS STRATEGY ■
Wean Yourself from Coffee

If you're a regular coffee drinker, you're probably familiar with the symptoms that occur when you don't get your daily dose. Caffeine withdrawal can cause an excruciating headache, as well as drowsiness and irritability. In extreme cases, nausea and vomiting can occur. For this reason, cold turkey may not be the best method to break your coffee habit. Here's a gentler method.

1. Begin to slowly cut your intake, at the rate of half a cup every day or two.
2. Plan ahead to substitute a healthy hot drink for your usual cup of coffee. Green tea is an excellent replacement, and it has a small amount of caffeine. You can also substitute BENEFICIAL herbal teas.
3. If you're accustomed to taking an afternoon coffee break, go for a brisk walk instead.
4. As you reduce your coffee intake, also begin to drink less coffee per cup—by making a weaker blend or adding soy milk.
5. Get plenty of rest!

Week 4

Blood Type Diet

- Continue at the week 3 level, focusing on BENEFICIAL and SUPER BENEFICIAL foods.

Exercise Regimen

- Continue at the week 3 level.
- Review your progress, noting in your journal improvements in strength and flexibility. Determine which exercise regimen has worked for you, including time of day, setting, and activity level.

■ **WEEK 4 SUCCESS STRATEGY** ■
Maximize Energy with the Right Eating Schedule

For Blood Type AB, the timing of your meals can be almost as important as what you eat. This is particularly true if you're trying to lose weight. The following are helpful guidelines:

- Never skip meals. You won't be "saving" calories, as the metabolic reaction will foil your efforts.
- Make breakfast your most important protein-rich meal of the day. The result will be an efficient metabolism all day long.
- Eat on a sliding scale: big breakfast, medium lunch, small dinner.
- Resist the late-night munchies, but if you have problems regulating blood sugar, have a small protein snack—yogurt or soy milk—before bedtime.

A Final Word

IN SUMMARY, the secret to fighting fatigue with the Blood Type AB Diet involves:

1. Maximizing overall health by eating a diet rich in soy protein, BENEFICIAL seafood, cultured dairy, and green vegetables.
2. Minimizing the consumption of toxic lectins, most abundant in chicken and in grains such as wheat, buckwheat, and corn.
3. Enhancing detoxification and elimination to increase liver efficiency and inhibit untoward provocation of the immune system by infectious agents.
4. Using supplements to improve digestive health, provide antioxidant support, and help balance immune function.

Appendices

A Simple Definition of Terms

agglutination: Clumping, or "gluing" together. One means by which the immune system defends against foreign matter and toxins, notably against lectins and opposing blood type material.

antibody: The product of the immune system when it is stimulated by specific antigens. There are many classes of antibodies, among them "agglutinins," which isolate foreign substances by clumping them together so that they may be eliminated. Blood Types O, A, and B manufacture antibodies to other blood types. Blood Type AB, the universal recipient, manufactures no antibodies to other blood types.

antigen: A chemical that provokes an immune system antibody response. The blood type "ID" present on the blood cells, identified as Type A or B, is one example. A Type AB cell has both of these antigens. The blood type having no antigen is described as O or "Zero." As we age, it is to our advantage to shore up our store of circulating anti-blood-type antigens, as lower levels mean increased susceptibility to diseases arising from substances and organisms bearing opposing antigens.

antioxidant: A substance known to moderate the oxidation, or aging, process in human cells, by lowering free radical levels. As cells function normally in the body, they produce damaged molecules— called free radicals. Antioxidants help prevent widespread cellular destruction by willingly donating components to stabilize free radicals. Many healthy foods are rich sources of antioxidants. Vitamins C, E, A, the element selenium, and many plants and plant-derived substances such as green tea, quercetin, larch arabinogalactan, and milk thistle are potent antioxidants.

autoimmune disease: Diseases generated when the cells that normally defend the body against infections mistakenly attack its own cells, tissues, and organs.

blood type: The term commonly used to refer to the ABO blood group system. Originally used primarily to determine suitable blood and organ donor–recipient matches, ABO type determines many of the digestive and immunological characteristics of the body, as well as susceptibility to the diseases arising from infection, immune suppression, and digestive impairment. It is also one of the tools of anthropology in establishing the origins, socioeconomic development, and movements of ancient peoples.

catecholamines: Adrenaline and noradrenaline, hormones released from the adrenal glands in response to stress.

cortisol: A catabolic hormone produced by the adrenal glands in response to trauma. Cortisol breaks down muscle tissue and converts the proteins from the tissue into energy.

cyclic AMP (cAMP): A cyclic nucleotide of adenosine that acts at the cellular level to regulate various metabolic processes and mediate the effects of many hormones.

dopamine: A neurochemical made deep inside the brain and projected to the frontal lobes. There is a strong association between the release of dopamine and reward or reinforcement of behavior. A dopamine imbalance is associated with a heightened reaction to stress and to several mental illnesses.

endotoxins: Part of the outer membrane of the cell wall of Gram-negative bacteria, such as *E. coli, Salmonella, Shigella, Pseudomonas, Neisseria, Haemophilus,* and other leading pathogens.

glutathione: A small molecule made inside almost every cell, from its three constituent amino acids: glycine, glutamate, and cysteine. Glutathione is the major antioxidant produced by the cell, protecting it from free radicals.

H-P-A Axis: The interplay of three endocrine glands—hypothalamus, pituitary, and adrenal—involved in a normal stress response.

hyperthyroidism: The overactive thyroid, conventionally treated with long-term anti-thyroid drugs or thyroidectomy, partial removal or destruction with radioactive iodine or surgery. Thyroid diseases show a preference for Blood Type O individuals. While medical intervention is recommended in the case of hyperthyroid function, reducing the types and amount of anti–blood type lectins present in the diet, especially those found in certain grains and legumes, can be of great help in resolving these conditions.

hypothyroidism: Underproduction of thyroid hormone, thyroxine (t3) and/or free triiodothyronine (t4). Conventionally treated by hormone replacement therapy. Thyroid conditions often respond favorably to a blood type–appropriate diet.

immune system: The physiological determination of and response to "self" and "non-self" accomplished through the action of many organs and cells throughout the body, essential to the preservation of its health and integrity.

lectins: Proteins that attach to preferred receptors in the human body. Food lectins are often blood type specific. A lectin's action may initiate agglutination, inflammation, the abnormal proliferation of cells of the immune and nervous systems, or insulin resistance, depending upon the type of cells targeted. Abundant in the vegetable kingdom, lectins are fewer in number and type among animal foods.

metabolism: The aggregate of physical and chemical processes by which organisms maintain life, in the opposing functions of building tissue (anabolism) and breaking down tissue and foreign matter to be used as fuel (catabolism).

mineralocorticoids: A group of hormones (the most important being aldosterone) that regulate the balance of water and electrolytes (ions such as sodium and potassium) in the body.

natural killer (NK) cells: A subset of T-lymphocyte cells that act as the first line of defense against infections and cancer cells.

nitric oxide (NO): A short-lived molecule crucial to the regulation of the central nervous system.

polyamines: A group of cell components (putrescine, spermidine, and spermine) that are important in the regulation of cell proliferation and cell differentiation. Although their exact functions have not yet been identified, it is clear that the polyamines play important roles in a number of cellular processes such as replication, transcription, and translation.

selectins: Proteins that mediate the binding of white blood cells to the walls of the blood vessels, signaling the initiation of the inflammatory response.

xenobiotics: Foreign chemicals found in the body. The word comes from *xenos*, meaning "foreign," and *bios*, meaning "life." Xenobiotics are found when the body absorbs chemicals that are not nutrients, or when normally occurring substances are modified from their natural molecular structures.

FAQs: Blood Type and Fatigue

I am Blood Type O and am three months pregnant. I get extremely sleepy in the afternoons and am really dragging by evening. What can I do to increase my energy?

Blood Type O relies on a diet high in animal protein (lean, organic cuts) and regular aerobic exercise, and these are both crucial for strength and energy. Exercise also helps to minimize nausea, which can cause nutrient deficiencies. If you are healthy and do not have a history of miscarriages, there is probably no reason why you can't continue your regular exercise program during the first trimester, but I'd suggest discussing this with your doctor.

My book for pregnant women, *Eat Right for Your Baby: The Individualized Guide to Fertility and Maximum Health During Pregnancy, Nursing, and Your Baby's First Year,* is now out in paperback. See appendix C for details.

I am undergoing chemotherapy treatments for breast cancer. The day after a treatment I can hardly get out of bed. Any suggestions? I'm Blood Type A.

Cancer-related fatigue (CRF) is one of the most common side effects of cancer and its treatment. In particular, cancer treatments often produce fatigue:

- **Chemotherapy** Any chemotherapy drug may cause fatigue, but it may be a more common side effect of drugs such as vincristine, vinblastine, and cisplatin.
- **Radiation therapy** Radiation therapy can cause cumulative fatigue (fatigue that increases over time). This can occur regardless of the treatment site. Fatigue usually lasts from three to four weeks after treatment stops but can continue for up to two to three months.
- **Bone marrow transplant** This aggressive form of treatment can cause fatigue that lasts up to one year.
- **Biological therapy** Interferons and interleukins are cytokines, natural cell proteins that are normally released by white blood cells in response to infection. These cytokines carry messages that regulate other elements of the immune and endocrine systems. In high amounts, these cytokines can be toxic and lead to persistent fatigue.
- **Decreased nutrition** from the side effects of treatments (such as nausea, vomiting, mouth sores, taste changes, heartburn, or diarrhea) can cause fatigue.
- **Anemia** from reduced blood counts can result from some cancer treatments, resulting in fatigue.
- **Medications** used to treat side effects such as nausea, pain, depression, anxiety, and seizures can cause fatigue.
- **Chronic, severe pain** increases fatigue.

During treatments, increase your compliance to the Blood Type Diet, practice soothing exercises such as yoga, and get plenty of rest.

I work in a hospital as a physical therapist and am constantly exposed to sick patients. A free flu shot is offered annually at this time to employees. Is it beneficial for me to be immunized or take my chances and risk becoming infected with the flu virus? I'm Type B.

You are probably better off with the flu (unless it's a lethal variant) as the protection from an actual case is more long-lasting, and Type Bs can get unusual vaccine reactions. Elderberry inhibits neuramidase, the enzyme used by the influenza virus to attach to the nose and throat, so perhaps a cup of elderberry tea before work would be a good idea.

Why are different exercises recommended for people with different blood types?

The exercise recommendations are focused on improving total systemic health, mainly the functioning of the organs, glands, and immune and circulatory systems of the body, as opposed to building muscle tissue (which can be viewed as a pleasant side effect). What strenuous exercise does for Type O, yoga does for Type A, and aerobic exercise does for Types B and AB. Exercise recommendations are made with a general bias toward a person with a sedentary lifestyle. The link between blood type, stress, and exercise is discussed in *Live Right 4 Your Type: The Individualized Prescription for Maximizing Health, Metabolism, and Vitality in Every Stage of Your Life.* See appendix C for details.

Can Type A drink wheatgrass juice?

The sprouting of wheat into wheatgrass destroys the lectin that is problematic in wheat. Sprouting also beneficially changes the nutrient profile of this grain, resulting in a nutrient-dense, enzyme-rich super food. Because of these factors, I consider wheatgrass to be an excellent addition to the diet for Blood Type A. As far as an amount, use your own judgment. Because of the concentrated nature of this food, a little goes a long way, so if you have not enjoyed wheatgrass juice before, start with a smaller amount.

I am a fifty-five-year-old Blood Type O woman with a long history of recurrent major depression. My naturopath has recommended

St. John's wort. Why do you discourage this supplement for Blood Type O?

Blood Type O has lower levels of the enzyme MAO, and St. John's wort is an MAO inhibitor. This may explain why many Type Os on St. John's wort say they feel "weird," or have disturbing dreams. I have found, however, that Blood Type Os with mild to moderate depression benefit from the amino acid tyrosine, which can boost dopamine levels, or the Russian adaptogenic herb rhodiola, which helps modulate adrenaline and dopamine levels in the brain.

Why do non-secretors have more fungal infections?

The increased susceptibility to fungal infections observed in non-secretors may be the result of several independent factors. First, it has been reported that non-secretors have lower levels of secretory IgA antibodies. These are the antibodies that reside in our saliva, vaginal fluid, etc., and protect our membranes. In addition, some evidence suggests that non-secretors have much more difficulty digesting simple sugars and carbohydrates. Recurrent vaginal yeast infections have been linked with a high carbohydrate content to the vaginal fluids, which has in turn been linked to a higher sugar/carbohydrate diet in some women.

I have pernicious anemia. Will iron supplements help?

Floridax, a liquid iron supplement, can be taken to increase iron levels, but it is very difficult for the body to absorb iron from food. Methylcobalamine (vitamin B_{12}) can be given by your physician via injection and should help raise the levels of iron in the system.

Two of my friends and I are Type As. We all started the Blood Type Diet at the same time, and after six weeks we had all lost around eight pounds. Since that time, a little over a month ago, none of us has lost any more weight. We are all concentrating on avoiding the foods that cause weight gain and including as much of the foods that help weight loss as possible. What are we doing wrong?

It is not uncommon for those just starting the diet to experience rapid and dramatic weight loss, followed by a "quiescent" period, where the weight loss slows down or stops completely. This is due to the fact that each individual can have several set points where the metabolic machinery (either for genetic or metabolic reasons) remains locked at a particular ratio of weight to body fat. Much of this is the result of the capacity of the body's insulin metabolism. Food lectins have been shown to compete with insulin on the body's fat cells.

Why is ghee so beneficial for Blood Types B and AB?

Ghee, also called clarified butter, sounds deadly to the arteries, but actually has a rather positive effect on the cholesterol and HDL (good cholesterol). In the intestines, ghee is converted to butyrate, a short-chain fatty acid that both regulates the intestinal flora and promotes the health of the colon tissue. This conversion is particularly efficient in Types B and AB. Ghee can be made at home or bought in health-food shops or Indian gourmet stores.

Should I avoid genetically engineered food?

Yes! Genetic engineering moves lectin molecules from one species to another. Since lectins are the molecules that interact with our blood types, an OK food can easily become an avoid. Currently, the only way to safely avoid "GE" foods is to choose organic.

Resources
and Products

General

Centers for Disease Control and Prevention
National Center for Infectious Diseases
Division of Viral and Rickettsial Diseases
Atlanta, GA 30333
404-639-1388 or 1-888-232-3228
http://www.cdc.gov/ncidod/diseases/cfs

American Autoimmune Related Diseases Association
22100 Gratiot Avenue
Detroit, MI 48201
586-776-3900
Web site: www.aarda.org

Broda O. Barnes Research Foundation
P.O. Box 110098
Trumbull, CT 06611
203-261-2101
Web site: www.brodabarnes.org

Environmental Research Foundation
P.O. Box 5036
Annapolis, MD 21403
410-263-1584
Web site: www.rachel.org

Thyroid Foundation of America
350 Ruth Sleeper Hall—RSL 350
Parkman Street
Boston, MA 02114
1-800-832-8321
Web site: www.tsh.org

American Academy of Allergy, Asthma and Immunology
611 East Wells Street
Milwaukee, WI 53202
1-800-822-ASMA (2762)
http://www.aaaai.org

Nutrition Research
The Institute for Human Individuality
Southwest College of Naturopathic Medicine
2140 E. Broadway Road
Tempe, AZ 85282
480-858-9100
Web site: www.ifhi-online.org

The Institute for Human Individuality is under the 501c3 status of Southwest College of Naturopathic Medicine. Its prime goal is to foster research in the expanding area of human nutrigenomics. Nutrigenomics seeks to provide a molecular understanding for how common dietary chemicals affect health by altering the expression or structure of an individual's genetic makeup. (IFHI is conducting currently a twelve-week random-ized, double-blind, controlled trial implementing the Blood Type Diet to determine its effects on the outcomes of patients with rheumatoid arthritis.)

Blood Type–Specific Resources

Dr. Peter D'Adamo

The D'Adamo Clinic in Wilton, Connecticut, blends time-honored natural healing techniques with state-of-the-art diagnostics. The clinic staff is comprised of naturopathic physicians (ND) working with medical doctors (MD), nurses (RN), and other licensed health professionals, all under the precepts and guidance of Dr. Peter D'Adamo. To find out more or to schedule an appointment, please contact:

The D'Adamo Clinic, LLC
213 Danbury Road
Wilton, CT 06897
203-834-7500

www.dadamo.com

The World Wide Web has proven to be a valuable venue for exploring and applying the tenets of the Blood Type Diet and lifestyle. Since January 1997, hundreds of thousands have visited the site to participate in the ABO chat groups, to peruse the scientific archives, to share experiences and recipes, and to learn more about the science of blood type.

Blood Type Specialty Products and Supplements

North American Pharmacal, Inc., is the official distributor of Blood Type specialty products. The product line includes supplements, books, tapes, teas, meal replacement bars, cosmetics, and support material that make eating and living right for your type easier.

North American Pharmacal, Inc.
12 High Street
Norwalk, CT 06851
Tel: 203-866-7664
Fax: 203-838-4066
Toll free: 877-ABO TYPE (877-226-8973)
www.4yourtype.com

Home Blood-Typing Kits

North American Pharmacal, Inc., is the official distributor of Home Blood Type Testing Kits. Each kit costs $9.95 (plus shipping and handling) and is a single-use, disposable, educational device capable of determining one individual's ABO and Rhesus (Rh) blood type. Results are obtained within about four to five minutes. If you have several friends or family members who need to learn their blood type, you will need to order a separate home blood-typing kit for each individual.

The Blood Type Library

The following books are available in bookstores, health-food stores, selected grocery and specialty stores, on the Web, and through North American Pharmacal.

Eat Right 4 Your Type
The Individualized Diet Solution to Staying Healthy, Living Longer, and Achieving Your Ideal Weight
By Dr. Peter J. D'Adamo, with Catherine Whitney
G. P. Putnam's Sons, 1996
The original Blood Type Diet book, with over two million copies sold in more than sixty-five languages.

Cook Right 4 Your Type
The Practical Kitchen Companion to Eat Right 4 Your Type
By Dr. Peter J. D'Adamo, with Catherine Whitney
G. P. Putnam's Sons, 1998 (Berkley Trade Paperback, 1999)
Includes over two hundred original recipes, thirty-day meal plans, and guidelines for each blood type.

Live Right 4 Your Type
The Individualized Prescription for Maximizing Health, Metabolism, and Vitality in Every Stage of Your Life
By Dr. Peter J. D'Adamo, with Catherine Whitney
G. P. Putnam's Sons, 2001
A total health and lifestyle plan based on the individual variations observed for each blood type. Includes new research on the mind-body connection and the importance of blood type secretor status.

Eat Right 4 Your Type Complete Blood Type Encyclopedia
By Dr. Peter J. D'Adamo, with Catherine Whitney
Riverhead Books, 2002
The A-to-Z reference guide for the blood type connection to symptoms, diseases, conditions, medications, vitamins, supplements, herbs, and food.

Right 4 Your Type Pocket Guides
Blood Type, Food, Beverage and Supplement Lists
By Peter J. D'Adamo, with Catherine Whitney
Berkley Books, 2002
The Eat Right 4 Your Type Portable and Personal Blood Type Guides are pocket-sized and user-friendly. They serve as a handy reference tool while shopping, cooking, and eating out. Each book contains the food, beverage, and supplement list for each blood type, plus handy tips and ideas for incorporating the Blood Type Diet into your daily life.

Eat Right 4 Your Baby
The Individualized Guide to Fertility and Maximum Health During Pregnancy, Nursing, and Your Baby's First Year
By Dr. Peter J. D'Adamo, with Catherine Whitney
G. P. Putnam's Sons, 2003

An invaluable guide for couples looking to combine the best of naturopathic and blood type science to maximize the health of mother and baby—with practical blood type–specific guidelines for achieving a healthy state before pregnancy, eating and living right during pregnancy, and continuing in good health during baby's first year.

Dr. Peter J. D'Adamo's Eat Right 4 (for) Your Type Health Library
Allergies: Fight Them with the Blood Type Diet ®
Arthritis: Fight It with the Blood Type Diet ®
Cancer: Fight It with the Blood Type Diet ®
Cardiovascular Disease: Fight It with the Blood Type Diet ®
Diabetes: Fight It with the Blood Type Diet ®

Index

Printed in the United States
by Baker & Taylor Publisher Services